ASSOCIATION OF PHYSICIANS INDIA

APICON 2025
Workshop Manual
Pulmonary Function Test

APICON 2025 Kolkata

APICON 2025
Workshop Manual
Pulmonary Function Test

Editors

Aloke Gopal Ghoshal
MD DNB FCCP Ex-WHO Fellow, Fellow ICS FICP
Medical Director
National Allergy Asthma Bronchitis Institute (NAABI)
Kolkata, West Bengal, India

Indranil Halder
MBBS DCH MD FRCP(Glasgow) FCCP(USA) FICP
European Diploma in Adult Respiratory Medicine
Associate Professor and Head
Department of Pulmonary Medicine
College of Medicine and JNM Hospital
Kalyani, West Bengal, India

JAYPEE

JAYPEE BROTHERS MEDICAL PUBLISHERS
The Health Sciences Publisher
New Delhi | London

JAYPEE **Jaypee Brothers Medical Publishers (P) Ltd**

Headquarters
EMCA House
23/23-B, Ansari Road, Daryaganj
New Delhi 110 002, India
Landline: +91-11-23272143, +91-11-23272703
+91-11-23282021, +91-11-23245672
E-mail: jaypee@jaypeebrothers.com

Corporate Office
Jaypee Brothers Medical Publishers (P) Ltd.
4838/24, Ansari Road, Daryaganj
New Delhi 110 002, India
Phone: +91-11-43574357
Fax: +91-11-43574314
E-mail: jaypee@jaypeebrothers.com

Overseas Office
JP Medical Ltd.
83, Victoria Street, London
SW1H 0HW (UK)
Phone: +44-20 3170 8910
Fax: +44(0)20 3008 6180
E-mail: info@jpmedpub.com

Website: www.jaypeebrothers.com
Website: www.jaypeedigital.com

Inquiries for bulk sales may be solicited at: jaypee@jaypeebrothers.com

APICON 2025 Workshop Manual Pulmonary Function Test / ***Aloke Gopal Ghoshal, Indranil Halder***

First Edition: **2025**

ISBN: 978-93-6616-417-5

Printed in India

Contributors

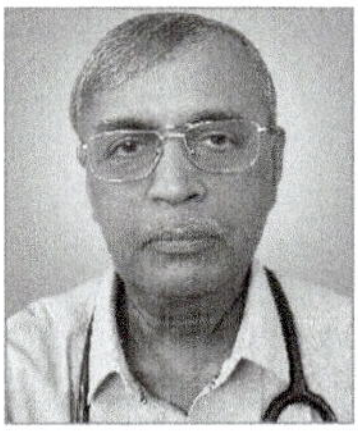

Aloke Gopal Ghoshal
MD DNB FCCP Ex-WHO Fellow, Fellow ICS FICP
Medical Director
National Allergy Asthma Bronchitis Institute (NAABI)
Kolkata, West Bengal, India

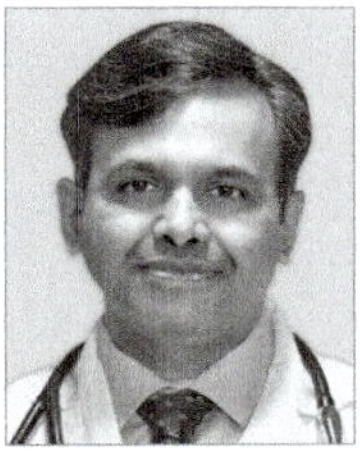

Indranil Halder
MBBS DCH MD FRCP(Glasgow) FCCP(USA) FICP
European Diploma in Adult Respiratory Medicine
Associate Professor and Head
Department of Pulmonary Medicine
College of Medicine and JNM Hospital
Kalyani, West Bengal, India

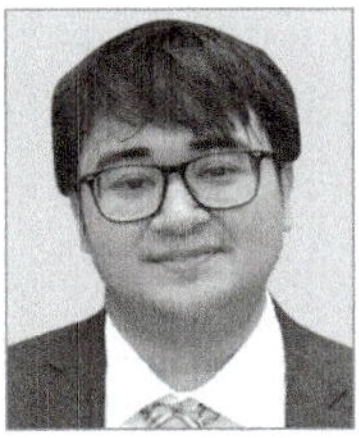

Arman Haque
MBBS FICC DNB[Respiratory Medicine (PGT)]
Postgraduate Trainee
Department of Pulmonary Medicine
College of Medicine and JNM Hospital
Kalyani, West Bengal, India

Preface

"Spirometry is an answer to a question"

The history of pulmonary function testing is a reflection of our understanding of the functioning of the respiratory system over the years. Our first stint with spirometry in the 70s was in the form of a huge drum submerged within water. It was a formidable sight, and the whole generation probably carried the awe and discomfort throughout their lifespan. The next generation witnessed the advent of computer-based spirometry in a handy set. However, the chief obstacle in popular acceptance persisted as effort dependence and variability of output. The current generation has been able to overcome the obstacles with impulse oximetry (does not need maximal effort), fractional exhaled nitric oxide (FeNO), and others. Still, spirometry remains underperformed and underutilized in our daily practice.

Pulmonary function test (PFT) is an elaborate and composite exercise. Office spirometry is the most common practiced version and apart from its clinical and epidemiological application is an academic exercise in itself. Interpretation needs thorough understanding of respiratory physiology as also reference values and interpretative standards.

John Hutchison is known to first coin the terms *spirometer* and *vital capacity* and understand the crucial role of spirometry in health and disease. The first standardization guidelines for spirometry were attempted from the American Thoracic Society (ATS) in 1979. Interpreting spirometry required the development of reference equations, and the first broadly adopted reference equations came from the European Coal and Steel Community in 1983. Standardization of spirometry provided the foundation for research at the global level, further establishing its role in clinical medicine. The oft-quoted Framingham study in the late 1960s showed a strong independent relationship between reduced forced vital capacity (FVC) and the risk of coronary heart disease. Several epidemiological studies followed including the National Health and Nutrition Examination Survey 1990 (NHANES) which corroborated the importance of spirometry as a risk factor for overall mortality, lung cancer, and cardiovascular disease.

The Fletcher and Peto study in the late 1970s demonstrated the progressive but variable lung function loss related to cigarette smoking. Spirometry got accepted as the basis of COPD diagnosis. Gradually, spirometry got wider application in the diagnosis of respiratory disease, monitoring disease status, assessing response to therapy, prognostication, preoperative assessment, and pulmonary research.

The technical parameters and quality control are of paramount importance in appropriate utilization of PFTs.

Interpretation involves three key aspects: (1) Classification of observed values for normal range with respect to a population of healthy individuals, (2) Integration of the knowledge of physiological determinants of test results into a functional classification of the identified impairments, and (3) Integration of the identified patterns with other clinical data to inform differential diagnosis and guide therapy. In 2005, the ATS and European Respiratory Society (ERS) jointly adopted technical standards for the interpretation of PFTs. In 2024, the 2005 recommendations were modified to establish the current standards for PFT interpretation.

Presently, spirometry is a safe noninvasive and affordable test incorporating emerging innovations in interpretation and performance. It a global health marker and may be amalgamated with other accepted health markers to add prognostic value. Spirometry can identify an increased risk of both respiratory and nonrespiratory disorders including cardiovascular and metabolic diseases. Spirometry has its utility at all ages throughout the lifespan, more so for the high-risk groups.

However, in spite of recognition of PFT as essential to respiratory disease diagnosis, management, and research, acceptance in primary and family care remains suboptimal. The crucial limitation of spirometry is its reliance on *forced* expiratory maneuvers. The lungs function naturally with tidal breathing and not with forced expiration. Effort dependence is always associated with variability and reproducibility concerns. Spirometry is often suboptimally performed by children or those with cognitive and physical impairment. It also fails to detect pathology until nearly 50% of small airways are affected and thus unable to accurately identify early respiratory disease affecting the small airways. Recently, concerns have been raised in spirometry interpretation incorporating ethnic reference equations.

Complementary technologies have emerged to assess lung function by respiratory oscillometry and others. Impulse oscillometry, first described by du Bois *et al.* in 1951, addresses some of the limitations of spirometry. Oscillometry involves applying small-pressure oscillations to the airway through application of multifrequency acoustic waves at the mouth at different frequencies and measuring how these oscillations are transmitted through the respiratory system. It assesses mechanical properties of the entire respiratory system, resulting in measurements of respiratory impedance. The most patient-friendly aspect of IOS is performance by tidal breathing. Oscillometry may provide accurate measurements across age ranges and in patients currently underserved by spirometry such as infants, the elderly, and those with physical or cognitive impairments. Oscillometry is also more sensitive than spirometry in the early diagnosis of COPD and assessing asthma control. Paucity of normal reference values for oscillometry is gradually being overcome by studies.

Measurement and monitoring of FeNO is a recent tool for clinical and epidemiological use. FeNO refers to the concentration of nitric oxide in exhaled breath expressed in parts per billion. NO is a key mediator involved in various physiological and pathological processes in the respiratory system. FeNO is more sensitive than spirometry at identifying type 2 airway inflammation in asthma and does not require forced expiratory maneuvers. Advances in FeNO measurement techniques have enhanced its utility, providing clinicians with a reliable tool to assess airway inflammation.

Lung clearance index from multiple breath inert gas washout is a promising alternative to spirometry with other technologies such as functional pulmonary magnetic resonance imaging and electrical impedance tomography.

Pulmonary function test is an execution of our understanding of respiratory physiology. Spirometry is an answer to a question. Quality control and infection-control measures are of paramount importance. Office spirometry, impulse oscillometry, and other parameters such as FeNO, DLCO, and body plethysmography are complementary to each other. PFT is yet to get proper recognition in clinical medicine.

Aloke Gopal Ghoshal
Indranil Halder

Contents

CHAPTER 1

Spirometry

INTRODUCTION

Spirometry is an important diagnostic and monitoring tool in pulmonary medicine, widely regarded as the foundation of respiratory assessment. By measuring the dynamics of airflow and lung volumes during forced breathing maneuvers, spirometry provides critical information about pulmonary function. Its simplicity, cost-effectiveness, and diagnostic utility make it a cornerstone in the evaluation of common respiratory disorders such as asthma, chronic obstructive pulmonary disease (COPD), and interstitial lung diseases (ILDs).

The 2024 American Thoracic Society (ATS) and European Respiratory Society (ERS) guidelines have introduced updated standards for spirometry performance, interpretation, and reporting. These updates emphasize improved reproducibility, standardization, and integration of technological advances. The role of spirometry extends beyond clinical practice, playing a significant part in occupational health evaluations, preoperative assessments, and clinical research.

BASICS OF SPIROMETRY

Definition

Spirometry is a pulmonary function test (PFT) designed to measure dynamic lung volumes and airflow rates. By capturing data during forced respiratory maneuvers, it provides quantitative insights into lung function, allowing clinicians to assess the presence, severity, and nature of respiratory impairment.

Key Parameters

According to the *2024 ATS/ERS guidelines*, the following parameters form the cornerstone of spirometric evaluation:

- *Forced vital capacity (FVC)*:
    - Definition: The total volume of air exhaled during a forced expiratory maneuver after maximal inhalation.
    - Clinical use: FVC is reduced in restrictive lung diseases and can also be diminished in severe obstructive conditions with air trapping.

- *Forced expiratory volume in 1 second (FEV_1)*:
  - Definition: The volume of air exhaled in the first second of the FVC maneuver.
  - Clinical use: A primary marker of airway obstruction, with reduced values seen in diseases such as COPD and asthma.
- *FEV_1/FVC ratio*:
  - Definition: The proportion of FVC expelled in the first second, expressed as a percentage.
  - Clinical use: A reduced ratio [less than lower limit of normal (LLN)] indicates obstructive ventilatory defects.
- *Peak expiratory flow (PEF)*:
  - Definition: The maximum flow achieved during a forced expiration.
  - Clinical use: Useful for detecting variable airway obstruction, especially in asthma.
- *Flow-volume loops*:
  - Definition: Graphical representation of flow against volume during the respiratory cycle.
  - Clinical use: Identifies characteristic patterns of obstruction (e.g., concavity in COPD) or upper airway abnormalities (e.g., flattening in variable extrathoracic obstruction).
- *Forced expiratory flow (FEF) 25–75%*:
  - Definition: The average flow rate during the middle portion of the FVC maneuver.
  - Clinical use: A marker for small airway dysfunction.

PHYSIOLOGICAL BASIS OF SPIROMETRY

Spirometry measures airflow and lung volumes, reflecting the mechanics of breathing:

- *Airflow resistance*: Assessed indirectly via changes in flow during forced exhalation.
- *Lung compliance*: Reflects the elastic properties of lung tissue and chest wall.
- *Airway caliber*: Changes in small and large airway diameters affect measured parameters, providing insights into diseases affecting these regions.

Updates in ATS/ERS 2024 Guidelines

The latest guidelines emphasize precision, standardization, and expanded applicability:

- *Acceptability criteria*: Revised criteria focus on ensuring high-quality maneuvers. Key elements include:
  - Absence of hesitation or false starts.
  - No coughing during the first second of exhalation.
  - A smooth, continuous effort throughout the maneuver.
  - Expiration lasting at least 6 seconds (3 seconds in children) or achieving a plateau.

- *Reproducibility standards*: At least three acceptable maneuvers are required, with the two best FVC and FEV_1 values differing by no more than:
  - 150 mL for adults.
  - 100 mL for children and individuals with predicted FVC < 1.0 L.
- *Reference equations*: Updated reference values incorporate global multi-ethnic datasets, enhancing accuracy in diverse populations.
- *Grading quality*: Tests are graded from A to F based on acceptability and reproducibility, with A indicating the highest quality.
- *Integration with digital tools*: Emphasis on using AI algorithms for automated detection of errors, quality control, and preliminary interpretation.

CLINICAL RELEVANCE

Spirometry is integral to evaluating:

- *Obstructive disorders*: Conditions such as COPD and asthma are characterized by airflow limitation, reflected by a reduced FEV_1/FVC ratio. Spirometry can differentiate between reversible and irreversible obstruction using bronchodilator response (BDR) testing.
- *Restrictive disorders*: Diseases like pulmonary fibrosis reduce lung volumes (e.g., FVC) while preserving or increasing the FEV_1/FVC ratio.
- *Mixed patterns*: Combined obstructive and restrictive patterns are seen in conditions like sarcoidosis or obesity-related hypoventilation.

TECHNIQUES AND EQUIPMENT

The accuracy and reliability of spirometry depend on both the equipment used and the methodology followed.

Types of Spirometers

Spirometers can be broadly categorized based on their operational principles and intended use.

Volume-displacement Spirometers

These devices measure lung volumes directly by recording the volume of air displaced during breathing maneuvers.

- Water-seal spirometers: The traditional gold standard, consisting of a bell immersed in a water chamber. While accurate, these devices are bulky and now mostly replaced by digital alternatives.
- Bellows spirometers: Utilize expandable bellows to measure volume. Like water-seal spirometers, they are less commonly used today.

Advantages

- High accuracy for volume measurements.
- Reliable in laboratory settings.

Disadvantages

- Bulky and not portable.
- Require regular maintenance.

Flow-sensing Spirometers (Pneumotachographs)

These devices measure airflow, which is then integrated over time to calculate lung volumes. Common types include:

- *Turbine spirometers*: Use a rotating vane or turbine to measure airflow. Simple and portable but less accurate at very high or low flow rates.
- *Ultrasonic spirometers*: Measure flow using sound waves. They are highly precise, require minimal calibration, and are unaffected by humidity or temperature changes.
- *Pressure differential spirometers*: Measure the pressure difference across a resistance to calculate flow.

Advantages

- Portable and user-friendly.
- Can integrate with digital systems for automated interpretation.

Disadvantages

- May require regular calibration and cleaning.
- Accuracy can be affected by high-resistance pathways or leaks.

Handheld or Portable Spirometers

Designed for screening and telemedicine, these compact devices provide rapid, basic spirometry data. However, they often lack advanced features required for full diagnostic evaluation.

METHODOLOGY

Pre-test Preparation

Proper preparation is critical for obtaining valid and reproducible spirometry results. The 2024 ATS/ERS guidelines outline the following steps:

- *Patient preparation*:
    - Understanding the procedure: Explain the test, emphasizing the importance of maximal effort and correct technique. Visual aids or demonstrations are helpful.
    - Avoidance of confounders:
        - No smoking, vigorous exercise, or large meals within 1–2 hours of the test.
        - Avoid using short-acting bronchodilators for at least 4 hours (unless bronchodilator response is being tested).
- *Equipment preparation*:
    - Calibration: Spirometers must be calibrated daily using a 3L calibration syringe, with volume accuracy maintained within ±3%.
    - Hygiene protocols: Disposable mouthpieces and anti-viral filters are recommended to minimize infection risks. Follow stringent cleaning guidelines for reusable components.
- *Environmental considerations*:
    - Test environment should be quiet, well-lit, and free from distractions.
    - Ensure ambient conditions (e.g., temperature and humidity) align with device specifications.

Steps of Performing Spirometry

Performing spirometry requires adherence to a standardized approach to ensure accuracy and reproducibility. The 2024 ATS/ERS guidelines emphasize both patient preparation and correct execution of the test.

Patient Positioning and Setup

Proper positioning is crucial for optimal lung expansion and consistent results.

Positioning

- *Seated position*:
  - The patient should sit upright with feet flat on the floor and legs uncrossed to prevent abdominal compression.
  - A straight posture minimizes thoracic restriction and ensures full lung expansion.
- *Head position*: The head should be slightly elevated and aligned to maintain a clear airway.

Use of a Nose Clip

- A nose clip prevents nasal airflow, ensuring that all air passes through the mouthpiece.
- If a nose clip is intolerable, patients must be instructed to breathe exclusively through their mouth.

Equipment Setup

- Ensure the spirometer is calibrated and a clean, disposable mouthpiece is attached.
- *Verify the test environment*: Avoid drafts, temperature fluctuations, and excessive noise.

Instruction and Demonstration

Clear communication with the patient is essential to achieve optimal effort during the test.

Pre-test Explanation

- Describe the purpose of the test and the steps involved.
- Emphasize the need for maximal inhalation and forceful, sustained exhalation.

Demonstration

- Demonstrate the procedure using the spirometer or a visual aid to build patient confidence.
- Highlight key points such as maintaining a tight seal on the mouthpiece and avoiding early termination of exhalation.

Performing the Maneuver

Step 1: Inhalation to Total Lung Capacity (TLC)

- Instruct the patient to inhale deeply until their lungs feel completely full.
- Encourage a quick and forceful transition to exhalation without hesitation.

Step 2: Forced Exhalation

- The patient should exhale as hard, fast, and completely as possible.
- Exhalation must continue until the flow has ceased or a plateau is achieved.
- Ensure that exhalation lasts at least 6 seconds in adults and 3 seconds in children (or until plateau).

Step 3: Reproducibility of Results

- Repeat the maneuver a minimum of three times, ensuring:
    - Two best FEV_1 and FVC values differ by no more than 150 mL for adults or 100 mL for children.
    - All efforts meet the acceptability criteria outlined below.

Quality Assurance

Acceptability Criteria (ATS/ERS 2024)

Each maneuver must meet the following conditions:

- *No hesitation at start*: The patient should avoid pausing or breathing erratically at the onset of exhalation.
- *Smooth and continuous effort*: The flow-volume loop should be free of erratic peaks or troughs.
- *No coughing during the first second*: Coughing or glottic closure can lead to underestimation of FEV_1.
- *Adequate exhalation time*: The maneuver should last ≥ 6 seconds in adults or until flow reaches < 25 mL/second for ≥ 1 second.
- *Tight seal around the mouthpiece*: Leakage leads to underreporting of lung volumes.

Reproducibility Criteria

Reproducibility ensures reliability of the test:

- At least two acceptable FEV_1 and FVC measurements must be within 150 mL (100 mL in children or low-volume patients).
- If reproducibility is not achieved within eight attempts, the test should be repeated after rest or rescheduled.

Common Errors and Corrections

Errors in Spirometry

- *Early termination*:
    - Result: Underestimation of FVC.
    - Correction: Reinforce the need for complete emptying of the lungs.
- *Submaximal effort*:
    - Result: Reduced FEV_1 and FVC.
    - Correction: Use motivational coaching and visual feedback (e.g., flow-volume curve).
- *Glottic closure or coughing*:
    - Result: Irregular flow-volume loop; inaccurate FEV_1.
    - Correction: Encourage relaxed but forceful breathing.

- *Air leak around the mouthpiece*:
  - Result: Invalid readings due to air escape.
  - Correction: Check mouthpiece seal and instruct patient to avoid biting or loosening their grip.

Grading of Test Quality

The 2024 ATS/ERS guidelines grade spirometry efforts from *A to F* based on the quality and reproducibility of results:

- *Grade A*: Three acceptable maneuvers, all within reproducibility criteria.
- *Grade B*: Three acceptable maneuvers, two within reproducibility criteria.
- *Grade C to F*: Fewer than three acceptable maneuvers or large variability in results.

Tests graded *C or lower* may be unreliable and should be interpreted with caution or repeated.

Post-test Protocol

Evaluation of Bronchodilator Response (if Indicated)

- Perform baseline spirometry, administer a short-acting bronchodilator (e.g., 400 μg salbutamol), and repeat the test after 15–20 minutes.
- A positive response is defined as an increase in FEV_1 or FVC ≥ 12% and ≥ 200 mL.

Data Review

- Ensure that results meet acceptability and reproducibility criteria.
- Cross-check flow-volume loops for artifacts or irregularities.

Feedback to Patient

Discuss the results briefly and address any concerns or discomfort experienced during the test.

Emerging Innovations in Spirometry Performance

- *Real-time feedback systems*: Modern spirometers provide visual and auditory cues during the maneuver, helping patients achieve optimal effort.
- *Telemedicine applications*: Portable spirometers with Bluetooth connectivity enable remote testing and real-time guidance from healthcare providers.
- *AI-assisted coaching*: AI tools analyze patient effort, identify errors, and provide tailored feedback to improve technique during the test.

INTERPRETATION OF SPIROMETRY

Interpretation of spirometry requires a structured approach to assess pulmonary function and identify obstructive, restrictive, or mixed ventilatory defects. Proper interpretation integrates clinical context, observed values, and reference standards. The 2024 ATS/ERS guidelines provide an updated framework for interpreting spirometric results with improved emphasis on precision, inclusivity of global reference equations, and alignment with evolving clinical applications.

Principles of Spirometry Interpretation

Stepwise Approach

- *Assess test quality*: Ensure the test meets acceptability and reproducibility criteria as outlined in the ATS/ERS 2024 guidelines.
- *Evaluate key parameters*:
  - FEV_1: Indicator of airway obstruction severity.
  - FVC: Reflects lung capacity and potential restriction.
  - FEV_1/FVC ratio: Critical for identifying obstruction.
- *Compare values to predicted norms*: Utilize updated reference equations tailored to the patient's demographic and physiological characteristics.
- *Classify the pattern of abnormality*: Determine if the defect is obstructive, restrictive, or mixed.
- *Correlate with clinical context*: Integrate spirometry findings with history, examination, and other investigations to confirm the diagnosis.

Key Diagnostic Patterns

Normal Spirometry

- *FEV_1/FVC ratio*: ≥ LLN.
- *FVC and FEV_1*: ≥ LLN.

Clinical implication: Normal spirometry does not rule out all pulmonary disorders (e.g., early interstitial lung disease or small airway dysfunction).

Obstructive Ventilatory Defect

- *Definition*: Reduced ability to expel air due to airway narrowing or obstruction.
- *Criteria*:
  - FEV_1/FVC ratio: < LLN.
  - FEV_1: Reduced (severity graded based on % predicted).
- *Grading of severity (ATS/ERS 2024)*: Refer to **Table 1**
- *Examples*:
  - Asthma: Obstruction with bronchodilator reversibility (≥ 12% and 200 mL increase in FEV_1 or FVC).
  - COPD: Persistent obstruction without significant reversibility.

Restrictive Ventilatory Defect

- *Definition*: Reduced lung volumes due to parenchymal or extrapulmonary processes.

TABLE 1: Grading of severity.

FEV_1 (% predicted)	Severity
≥ 80%	Mild
50–79%	Moderate
30–49%	Severe
< 30%	Very severe

- *Criteria*:
  - FEV_1/FVC ratio: Normal or increased.
  - FVC: < LLN.
- *Confirmation*: Restriction must be confirmed by additional tests [e.g., total lung capacity (TLC) via plethysmography].
- *Examples*:
  - Interstitial lung diseases (e.g., idiopathic pulmonary fibrosis).
  - Neuromuscular disorders (e.g., myasthenia gravis).

Mixed Ventilatory Defect

- *Definition*: Combined features of obstruction and restriction.
- *Criteria*:
  - FEV_1/FVC ratio: < LLN.
  - FVC: < LLN.
  - TLC: Reduced (to confirm restriction).
- *Examples*:
  - Sarcoidosis.
  - Combined COPD and obesity-related restrictive patterns.

Reference Values and Lower Limit of Normal

Updated Reference Equations (2024 ATS/ERS Guidelines)

- *Global multiethnic reference data*:
  - Incorporates population diversity to improve accuracy across different ethnicities.
  - Variables include age, sex, height, weight, and ethnicity.
- *Defining abnormality*:
  - Lower limit of normal: Defined as the 5th percentile of a healthy population. Values below this are considered abnormal.
  - Fixed-ratio cutoffs (e.g., $FEV_1/FVC < 0.70$) are now de-emphasized due to their limitations in older adults and certain ethnic groups.

Advanced Concepts in Interpretation

Bronchodilator Response Testing

- *Purpose*: Distinguish between reversible and irreversible airway obstruction.
- *Methodology*: Perform spirometry before and 15–20 minutes after administering a short-acting bronchodilator.
- *Positive response*: Increase in FEV_1 or FVC $\geq 12\%$ and ≥ 200 mL.

Flow-volume Loop Analysis

- *Key features*:
  - Obstruction: Concave expiratory limb (e.g., COPD and asthma).
  - Restriction: Proportional reduction in both inspiratory and expiratory volumes, with narrow loops.
  - Upper airway obstruction: Flattening of inspiratory and/or expiratory limbs (e.g., tracheal stenosis).

Small Airway Dysfunction

FEF 25–75% is a sensitive marker for small airway impairment, often seen in early asthma or environmental exposure-related lung injury.

Severity Indexing

Severity should be contextualized with symptoms, clinical findings, and comorbidities rather than relying solely on numerical thresholds.

Integration with Clinical Context

- *Occupational and environmental medicine*: Spirometry plays a key role in surveillance programs for workers exposed to airborne hazards (e.g., silica, asbestos). Early detection of abnormalities facilitates timely intervention.
- *Preoperative assessment*: Spirometry identifies patients at risk of postoperative complications, particularly in abdominal or thoracic surgeries.
- *Epidemiological research*: Population-based spirometry data provide insights into the burden and progression of lung diseases globally.

Reporting Standards

The 2024 ATS/ERS guidelines emphasize structured, comprehensive reports:

- *Patient information*: Demographics, clinical history, and test conditions.
- *Spirometry data*: Absolute and percent-predicted values for FEV_1, FVC, FEV_1/FVC, and other key metrics.
- *Interpretation*: Summary of findings (e.g., "moderate obstructive defect with bronchodilator response").
- *Graphical representation*: Flow-volume curves and volume-time graphs for visual assessment.
- *Quality grading*: Report the test quality (e.g., A to F) and any limitations affecting reliability.

PRECAUTIONS IN PERFORMING SPIROMETRY

Patient Factors

- *Understanding and cooperation*:
  - Patients must be fully informed about the procedure. Misunderstanding or anxiety can lead to suboptimal effort or incomplete maneuvers.
  - Demonstrating the test before performance can significantly enhance cooperation.
- *Medical conditions*:
  - Avoid spirometry during acute respiratory infections (e.g., viral bronchitis) as it may exacerbate symptoms and distort results.
  - Be cautious in patients with cardiovascular instability, recent surgeries, or severe dyspnea.
- *Pre-test restrictions*:
  - Ensure the patient refrains from smoking, consuming caffeine, or engaging in vigorous exercise for at least 2 hours before the test.

    - Suspend short-acting bronchodilators 4–6 hours before testing unless the bronchodilator response is being assessed.
- *Special populations*:
    - Children: Adapt instructions to their level of understanding, and use pediatric-specific reference values.
    - Elderly: Take into account reduced muscle strength and slower reaction times, which may affect results.
    - Obesity: Recognize that reduced chest wall compliance may mimic a restrictive pattern.

Equipment and Environment

- *Calibration and maintenance*:
    - Calibrate the spirometer daily using a 3 L syringe to ensure volume accuracy within ±3%.
    - Periodically verify flow sensor performance to detect deviations caused by wear or debris accumulation.
- *Hygiene protocols*:
    - Use disposable mouthpieces with integrated filters to minimize cross-contamination.
    - Follow stringent cleaning guidelines for reusable components between patients.
- *Environmental conditions*:
    - Conduct the test in a quiet, temperature-controlled room free from strong air currents.
    - Ensure ambient temperature, humidity, and barometric pressure are within the acceptable range specified by the spirometer manufacturer.

Common Pitfalls and How to Avoid them?

Patient-related Errors

- *Submaximal effort*:
    - Issue: Results in underestimation of FEV_1 and FVC.
    - Solution: Provide clear, enthusiastic coaching and use real-time graphical feedback.
- *Early termination of exhalation*:
    - Issue: Leads to an incomplete FVC measurement.
    - Solution: Emphasize the need for complete lung emptying; repeat the maneuver if exhalation is < 6 seconds in adults.
- *Coughing during the test*:
    - Issue: Creates flow interruptions, particularly during the first second, affecting FEV_1.
    - Solution: If coughing occurs, discard the attempt and provide feedback on maintaining a steady effort.
- *Leakage around the mouthpiece*:
    - Issue: Results in air loss, leading to falsely low readings.

- Solution: Ensure a tight seal; check for biting or improper positioning of the mouthpiece.

- *Poor coordination*:
  - Issue: Hesitation between inhalation and exhalation leads to an unsteady flow-volume curve.
  - Solution: Reinforce the importance of transitioning quickly from maximum inhalation to forced exhalation.

Equipment-related Errors

- *Inadequate calibration*:
  - Issue: Drift in calibration affects accuracy, especially for flow-sensing spirometers.
  - Solution: Calibrate daily and after any suspected deviation in performance.
- *Faulty sensors or tubing*:
  - Issue: Blocked or damaged sensors introduce errors in flow or volume measurements.
  - Solution: Regularly inspect and maintain spirometer components.
- *Incorrect software settings*:
  - Issue: Misconfigured demographic data (e.g., age, height, and ethnicity) result in incorrect predicted values.
  - Solution: Double-check patient details entered into the spirometer software.

Interpretation Pitfalls

- *Over-reliance on fixed ratios*:
  - Issue: Using a fixed FEV_1/FVC cutoff (e.g., 0.70) can misclassify obstruction, particularly in older adults or certain ethnic groups.
  - Solution: Use the LLN based on age- and ethnicity-adjusted reference equations.
- *Neglecting clinical context*:
  - Issue: Isolated spirometry results may not reflect the true underlying pathology.
  - Solution: Always integrate spirometry findings with clinical history, examination, and additional investigations.
- *Ignoring flow-volume loops*:
  - Issue: Significant diagnostic clues (e.g., upper airway obstruction) may be missed.
  - Solution: Routinely evaluate both numerical data and graphical outputs.
- *Failure to account for variability*:
  - Issue: Variations in repeated spirometry efforts can indicate technical errors or inconsistent patient effort.
  - Solution: Insist on reproducibility (FEV_1 and FVC within 150 mL for adults).

Safety Considerations in Special Scenarios

Bronchodilator Administration

- Monitor for adverse effects such as tremors, palpitations, or paradoxical bronchospasm during post-bronchodilator testing.
- Use standardized doses and delivery methods (e.g., metered-dose inhaler with spacer).

Exercise-induced Spirometry

- Ensure a controlled environment to prevent hyperventilation or exercise-induced bronchospasm.
- Provide adequate recovery time between maneuvers.

Postoperative and High-risk Patients

- Avoid spirometry if there is a high risk of complications (e.g., post-thoracic surgery, acute myocardial infarction).
- Conduct tests under close monitoring in high-risk cases.

ADVANCED CONCEPTS IN SPIROMETRY

Advanced applications of spirometry extend beyond routine diagnostic assessments. These concepts cater to complex clinical scenarios, research applications, and specialized populations.

Small Airway Function and Early Disease Detection

Forced Expiratory Flow at 25–75%

- *Definition*: FEF 25–75% measures the flow rate in the mid-portion of forced exhalation, reflecting small airway patency.
- *Clinical relevance*:
  - Sensitive indicator of small airway dysfunction in asthma, early COPD, and exposure-related lung injury.
  - Abnormal FEF 25–75% may precede changes in FEV_1 and FVC, identifying early disease.
- *Limitations*: High variability and dependency on FVC make FEF 25–75% a supportive, rather than definitive, diagnostic tool.

Oscillometry

Used in conjunction with spirometry, oscillometry evaluates small airways by measuring respiratory system impedance. This emerging tool is particularly valuable for patients unable to perform forced maneuvers.

Flow-volume Loop Analysis

Flow-volume loops provide graphical insights into airway dynamics, complementing numerical spirometry results.

Interpretation of Flow-volume Loop Patterns

Refer to **Table 2**.

Longitudinal Monitoring and Disease Progression

Serial Spirometry

- *Purpose*: Monitor lung function changes over time in chronic diseases (e.g., COPD, and cystic fibrosis).
- *Key metrics*:
  - Annual decline in FEV_1 is a marker of disease progression, particularly in obstructive lung diseases.
  - Rapid decline (> 40 mL/year) indicates poor disease control or accelerated progression.

Response to Therapy

Spirometry evaluates treatment efficacy, especially after interventions such as bronchodilators, anti-inflammatory therapies, or pulmonary rehabilitation.

Advanced Spirometry Applications

Preoperative Assessment

- Spirometry predicts perioperative risk, particularly for thoracic, abdominal, and cardiac surgeries.
- Patients with an FEV_1 < 50% predicted or significant obstruction/restriction are at higher risk for postoperative complications.

Occupational and Environmental Lung Disease

- *Surveillance programs*: Monitor lung function in workers exposed to respiratory hazards (e.g., miners, factory workers).

TABLE 2: Describing the flow-volume loop patterns with examples.

Pattern	Description	Examples
Normal loop	Symmetric inspiratory and expiratory curves; peak flow reached early in exhalation	Healthy individuals
Obstruction (e.g., COPD)	Concave expiratory limb; reduced peak expiratory flow	COPD, and asthma
Restriction	Narrow loop with proportional reduction in inspiratory and expiratory volumes	Interstitial lung disease
Fixed upper airway obstruction	Flattening of both inspiratory and expiratory limbs, indicating constant airflow limitation	Tracheal stenosis
Variable extrathoracic obstruction	Flattened inspiratory curve with preserved expiratory peak flow	Vocal cord dysfunction
Variable intrathoracic obstruction	Flattened expiratory curve with preserved inspiratory peak flow	Tracheomalacia

- *Early detection*: Spirometry identifies subclinical impairments, prompting interventions to prevent progression.

Emerging Trends in Spirometry

Global Lung Initiative Equations

- The 2024 ATS/ERS guidelines endorse the use of global lung initiative (GLI) reference equations for global standardization.
- GLI incorporates multiethnic, age, and gender-specific data, addressing disparities in diagnostic thresholds.

Integration with AI

AI algorithms improve interpretation accuracy by analyzing flow-volume loops, detecting subtle abnormalities, and grading test quality in real time.

Portable and Home Spirometry

- Advances in miniaturized, bluetooth-enabled spirometers facilitate remote monitoring of patients with chronic lung diseases.
- Real-time data sharing with clinicians enables early intervention for exacerbations.

ADVANCED INTERPRETATION IN SPECIAL POPULATIONS

Pediatrics

- Pediatric spirometry requires modifications in technique and interpretation.
- *Challenges*: Smaller airways, limited cooperation, and need for child-specific reference equations.

Geriatrics

- Aging affects lung elasticity, leading to reduced FEV_1 and FVC even in healthy elderly individuals.
- Reference equations incorporating age-related changes are essential for accurate interpretation.

Athletes

Highly trained athletes may exhibit high FVC values and near-normal or mildly reduced FEV_1/FVC ratios, complicating differentiation from pathological patterns.

FUTURE DIRECTIONS

Integration with Genomics and Biomarkers

Combining spirometry with genetic and molecular data may enable personalized respiratory medicine.

Remote Monitoring Ecosystems

Cloud-based spirometry integrated with wearable technology can track real-time lung function in chronic disease management.

Global Health Initiatives

- Expanding access to spirometry in low-resource settings through cost-effective, portable devices and telemedicine platforms.

CHAPTER

2

Fractional Exhaled Nitric Oxide

INTRODUCTION

The measurement of fractional exhaled nitric oxide (FeNO) has become a pivotal non-invasive biomarker in the evaluation and management of respiratory diseases, particularly asthma. Nitric oxide (NO) is a key mediator involved in various physiological and pathological processes in the respiratory system. Advances in FeNO measurement techniques have enhanced its utility, providing clinicians with a reliable tool to assess airway inflammation. Recent guidelines the European Respiratory Society (ERS), American Thoracic Society (ATS), and British Thoracic Society (BTS), have refined the indications and interpretation of FeNO, establishing its role in precision medicine for respiratory care.

What is FeNO?

FeNO refers to the concentration of NO in the exhaled breath, expressed in parts per billion (ppb). NO is synthesized from L-arginine by nitric oxide synthases (NOSs) in the epithelial cells of the respiratory tract. The primary source of FeNO in the airways is inducible nitric oxide synthase (iNOS), which is upregulated in response to inflammatory cytokines, particularly in type 2 inflammation.

FeNO measurement is standardized, with the ATS and ERS defining protocols for the technique. The device captures exhaled air at a controlled flow rate, minimizing contamination from nasal NO and ensuring reproducible results. Elevated FeNO levels are strongly associated with eosinophilic airway inflammation, making it a surrogate marker for this phenotype of inflammation. FeNO also serves as an indicator of corticosteroid responsiveness, playing a critical role in guiding anti-inflammatory therapies.

Why is it Done?

FeNO measurement serves as a biomarker for type 2 airway inflammation and is primarily used in the diagnosis and management of asthma. The technique offers insights into:

- *Airway inflammation*: FeNO quantifies eosinophilic inflammation, allowing differentiation from non-eosinophilic asthma phenotypes.

- *Treatment response*: It helps evaluate the effectiveness of corticosteroid therapy, with reductions in FeNO indicating a positive response.
- *Monitoring*: Regular FeNO assessments guide long-term asthma management, aiding in dose adjustment and predicting exacerbations.
- *Phenotyping*: It assists in identifying patients likely to benefit from targeted biologic therapies.
- *Prognostication*: FeNO levels are predictive of asthma exacerbations, particularly in poorly controlled asthma.
- *Research applications*: FeNO is widely used as a biomarker in clinical trials for new asthma therapies, enabling precise evaluation of anti-inflammatory treatments.

Indications

The clinical indications for FeNO measurement are outlined in guidelines from ERS, ATS, and BTS, emphasizing its use in the following scenarios:

- *Diagnosis of asthma*: FeNO supports the identification of eosinophilic airway inflammation, particularly in patients with atypical or inconclusive spirometry findings. High FeNO levels can distinguish eosinophilic asthma from other forms of airway diseases, such as COPD or non-eosinophilic asthma.
- *Prediction of corticosteroid responsiveness*: Elevated FeNO levels predict a favorable response to inhaled corticosteroids (ICS). This prediction can guide clinicians in choosing appropriate anti-inflammatory therapies.
- *Monitoring of asthma control*: Serial FeNO measurements aid in assessing treatment adherence, response, and the need for dose adjustments. Reductions in FeNO are indicative of effective anti-inflammatory control.
- *Differentiation of asthma phenotypes*: FeNO differentiates eosinophilic asthma from other phenotypes such as neutrophilic asthma, aiding in precise phenotyping for targeted therapy.
- *Guiding biologic therapy*: In patients eligible for biologics targeting type 2 inflammation (e.g., anti-IL-5, anti-IL-13 therapies), FeNO levels provide an additional biomarker for patient selection. High FeNO levels often correlate with elevated blood eosinophil counts and periostin levels, indicative of type 2 inflammation.
- *Assessment of occupational asthma*: FeNO testing identifies eosinophilic inflammation in workers exposed to occupational allergens, assisting in early diagnosis and intervention.
- *Assessment of comorbidities*: FeNO is increasingly being used in conditions with overlapping type 2 inflammation, such as allergic rhinitis (AR) and eosinophilic bronchitis, ensuring comprehensive airway management.

Utility

The utility of FeNO spans across diagnostic, therapeutic, and prognostic domains:

- *Diagnosis*: FeNO augments traditional diagnostic tools like spirometry and peak flow monitoring by identifying type 2 inflammation. According to ATS guidelines, FeNO values above 50 ppb in adults (and 35 ppb in children) are strongly suggestive of eosinophilic inflammation. These thresholds have high sensitivity and specificity for identifying corticosteroid-responsive asthma.

- *Therapeutic guidance*: FeNO directs the use of ICS, optimizing dose titration and minimizing overtreatment. A significant reduction in FeNO (often defined as >20% decrease) after initiating corticosteroids is a reliable marker of treatment effectiveness.
- *Prediction of exacerbations*: Elevated FeNO levels correlate with an increased risk of asthma exacerbations, making it a predictive tool for preventive strategies. Studies have shown that FeNO-guided treatment plans significantly reduce the frequency of exacerbations in patients with poorly controlled asthma.
- *Assessment of adherence*: A persistently elevated FeNO despite prescribed ICS therapy may indicate poor adherence, inadequate delivery, or alternative sources of airway inflammation. Real-time feedback using FeNO can improve patient adherence and therapeutic outcomes.
- *Research*: FeNO serves as a biomarker in clinical trials, evaluating novel therapeutics targeting airway inflammation. It provides quantitative endpoints for assessing the efficacy of biologic therapies, such as dupilumab and mepolizumab.
- *Monitoring in children*: FeNO is particularly valuable in pediatric populations, where invasive tests may not be feasible. It provides an objective measure of airway inflammation, guiding early intervention and long-term asthma control.

Procedure

FeNO measurement is a straightforward, noninvasive procedure performed using a portable or stationary device. The ATS/ERS standardized protocol includes:

- *Preparation*: Patients should avoid eating, drinking, smoking, or exercising for at least one hour before the test. Certain medications, such as ICS, leukotriene receptor antagonists, or nasal decongestants, can affect FeNO levels and should be withheld as clinically appropriate.
- *Technique*:
  - The patient inhales deeply to total lung capacity and then exhales steadily into the device at a controlled flow rate (50 mL/s).
  - The exhalation should last 6 seconds in adults and 4 seconds in children.
- *Repeatability*: At least two measurements within 5% or 2 ppb of each other are required to ensure accuracy. Additional measurements may be needed in cases of variability or patient non-compliance.
- *Device calibration*: Modern FeNO analyzers are designed for minimal calibration requirements, but periodic checks against standard NO concentrations are recommended to ensure accuracy.
- *Interpretation*: FeNO values are analyzed against established reference ranges, adjusted for age, height, and atopy. These values are interpreted in conjunction with clinical symptoms, spirometry, and other diagnostic findings.

Issues and Interpretation

Despite its utility, FeNO measurement has limitations and requires careful interpretation:

- *Variability*: FeNO levels are influenced by multiple factors, including age, sex, smoking status, atopy, and recent infections. Smokers typically exhibit lower FeNO levels due to NO scavenging effects of cigarette smoke, which may obscure underlying inflammation.
- *Non-asthmatic elevation*: Elevated FeNO can occur in other conditions, such as AR, eczema, or eosinophilic bronchitis, necessitating a comprehensive clinical correlation. Additionally, systemic inflammatory diseases and certain viral infections may transiently increase FeNO levels.
- *Low FeNO despite inflammation*: Conditions like neutrophilic asthma or recent corticosteroid use can result in low FeNO levels despite ongoing airway inflammation. Such cases require alternative markers, such as sputum eosinophil counts or exhaled breath condensate analysis, for accurate assessment.
- *Device standardization*: Differences in devices and calibration methods may affect FeNO readings. Adherence to ATS/ERS protocols is essential to minimize variability across different clinical settings.
- *Cost and accessibility*: The availability of FeNO devices and the associated costs may limit widespread use in resource-constrained settings. Portable devices have improved accessibility but remain expensive for routine use.
- *Emerging challenges*: Novel applications of FeNO, such as in interstitial lung diseases and pulmonary hypertension, require further research to establish their clinical relevance.

Interpretation Guidelines (ATS/ERS)

- *Low FeNO (<25 ppb in adults; <20 ppb in children)*: Unlikely to indicate eosinophilic inflammation. Alternative diagnoses or phenotypes should be considered.
- *Intermediate FeNO (25–50 ppb in adults; 20–35 ppb in children)*: Possible eosinophilic inflammation; clinical correlation required.
- *High FeNO (>50 ppb in adults; >35 ppb in children)*: Strongly suggestive of eosinophilic inflammation and corticosteroid responsiveness. High FeNO values also correlate with increased expression of IL-13 and periostin in the airway epithelium, hallmark features of type 2 inflammation.

Confounders of FeNO: Falsely Elevated and Reduced Values

Falsely Elevated FeNO Values

Several factors can lead to elevated FeNO levels that do not necessarily indicate airway inflammation, requiring careful interpretation in the clinical context:

- *Allergic rhinitis*: Elevated FeNO is often observed in patients with AR due to upper airway inflammation. Nasal NO contributes to higher readings, particularly if nasal NO contamination occurs during measurement.

- *Eosinophilic esophagitis and gastroesophageal reflux disease (GERD)*: These conditions can cause systemic eosinophilia or alter airway inflammation, leading to falsely elevated FeNO.
- *Environmental influences*: Exposure to allergens or high ambient NO levels, such as in polluted areas, can transiently elevate FeNO levels.
- *Dietary Factors*: High intake of nitrates, such as in green leafy vegetables or beetroot, can increase systemic NO production, indirectly affecting FeNO levels.
- *Non-asthmatic respiratory conditions*: Conditions like eosinophilic bronchitis or systemic inflammatory diseases, including vasculitides, may present with elevated FeNO without significant airway obstruction.
- *Recent upper respiratory tract infections*: Viral infections can temporarily increase FeNO due to heightened immune responses and airway epithelial activation.

Falsely Reduced FeNO Values

Conversely, several factors can suppress FeNO levels, potentially masking underlying airway inflammation:

- *Smoking*: Tobacco smoke has a well-documented inhibitory effect on NO production by airway epithelial cells. Smokers often exhibit reduced FeNO, even in the presence of type 2 inflammation.
- *Use of corticosteroids*: Recent use of inhaled or systemic corticosteroids significantly suppresses FeNO by downregulating iNOS expression, potentially yielding low levels despite underlying inflammation.
- *Neutrophilic airway inflammation*: Non-eosinophilic asthma phenotypes, characterized by neutrophilic inflammation, typically do not produce elevated FeNO, limiting its diagnostic utility in these cases.
- *Airway obstruction*: Severe airway obstruction or altered ventilation-perfusion ratios, as seen in advanced COPD or asthma, can reduce FeNO levels by limiting NO exhalation.
- *Systemic conditions*: Conditions like cystic fibrosis or primary ciliary dyskinesia, associated with altered airway epithelial function, may result in low FeNO despite coexisting inflammation.
- *Medications*: Nonsteroidal anti-inflammatory drugs (NSAIDs) or leukotriene receptor antagonists may impact FeNO levels by modulating inflammatory pathways.
- *Poor technique or compliance*: Inadequate exhalation or improper use of FeNO measurement devices can artifactually lower readings, underscoring the importance of standardized protocols.

Clinical Implications of Confounders

Understanding these confounders is critical for accurate FeNO interpretation. A comprehensive clinical assessment, including correlation with symptoms, spirometry, and other biomarkers, is essential to contextualize FeNO readings. Additionally, adherence to standardized ATS/ERS measurement protocols and awareness of individual patient factors, such as comorbidities and medication use, can help mitigate the impact of confounders, ensuring precise and reliable application of FeNO in clinical practice.

Role of FeNO in Allergic Rhinitis

Allergic rhinitis is a prevalent condition characterized by nasal inflammation mediated by immunoglobulin E (IgE) in response to allergen exposure. Although primarily affecting the upper airways, AR often coexists with asthma, reflecting the concept of the unified airway. FeNO measurement has emerged as a useful tool in evaluating type 2 inflammation in AR, highlighting its role in this broader spectrum of respiratory diseases.

PATHOPHYSIOLOGY LINKING FeNO AND ALLERGIC RHINITIS

Nitric oxide plays a pivotal role in the pathophysiology of AR. In AR, allergens stimulate the production of inflammatory cytokines such as interleukin (IL)-4, IL-5, and IL-13, which drive type 2 inflammation. IL-13, in particular, upregulates iNOS in the respiratory epithelium, leading to increased NO production. While nasal NO is primarily localized to the upper airways, a significant overlap exists between nasal and bronchial inflammation in AR patients, contributing to elevated FeNO levels.

CLINICAL UTILITY OF FeNO IN ALLERGIC RHINITIS

FeNO provides a non-invasive biomarker for assessing airway inflammation in AR. Its utility spans diagnostic, monitoring, and therapeutic domains:

- *Detection of subclinical lower airway involvement*:
    - AR often precedes or coexists with asthma, with shared inflammatory pathways. FeNO can identify subclinical lower airway inflammation in AR patients, aiding in early detection of asthma or predisposition to it.
    - Studies have demonstrated higher FeNO levels in AR patients with concomitant asthma compared to those with AR alone, underscoring its value in phenotyping disease overlap.
- *Correlation with disease severity*:
    - Elevated FeNO levels correlate with AR severity, particularly in patients with perennial or poorly controlled AR.
    - FeNO can reflect the inflammatory burden in AR, providing an objective measure of disease activity.
- *Guiding anti-inflammatory therapy*:
    - FeNO serves as a marker for corticosteroid responsiveness in AR patients. Reductions in FeNO after initiating intranasal or systemic corticosteroids indicate effective suppression of type 2 inflammation.
    - It helps identify patients who may benefit from additional anti-inflammatory therapies, particularly those with overlapping asthma or recalcitrant symptoms.

- *Predicting treatment outcomes*: In AR patients receiving allergen immunotherapy (AIT), FeNO trends can serve as a biomarker for treatment efficacy, reflecting reductions in type 2 inflammation over time.
- *Monitoring comorbidities*:
  - FeNO provides insights into the coexistence of asthma in AR patients, guiding comprehensive management strategies.
  - Elevated FeNO in AR patients may prompt further evaluation for lower airway involvement, ensuring early intervention and improved outcomes.

FeNO AND THE UNIFIED AIRWAY CONCEPT

The unified airway concept posits that the upper and lower respiratory tracts are anatomically and functionally interconnected. AR-induced inflammation can affect bronchial airways, resulting in elevated FeNO. Studies have shown:

- AR patients exhibit higher FeNO levels compared to healthy controls, even in the absence of clinically apparent asthma.
- Effective treatment of AR, such as with intranasal corticosteroids or antihistamines, can reduce FeNO levels, suggesting amelioration of systemic airway inflammation.
- FeNO-guided interventions in AR can potentially prevent progression to asthma, particularly in high-risk populations.

CONCLUSION

FeNO has emerged as an indispensable tool in the management of respiratory diseases, offering a precise, non-invasive method to assess airway inflammation. Its integration into clinical practice complements traditional diagnostic modalities, enabling personalized asthma management. However, appropriate training, adherence to standardized protocols, and judicious interpretation are critical for maximizing its clinical utility. Future advancements may further enhance its application, broadening the scope of FeNO beyond asthma to other inflammatory airway diseases. Additionally, continued research into the molecular pathways driving NO production will likely yield novel therapeutic targets, reinforcing its central role in respiratory medicine.

CHAPTER 3

Impulse Oscillometry

INTRODUCTION TO IMPULSE OSCILLOMETRY

Historical Background and Development

Impulse oscillometry (IOS) is a non-invasive pulmonary function test developed to measure airway resistance and reactance. The technique utilizes oscillatory pressure signals to assess mechanical properties of the respiratory system. The early conceptualization of forced oscillation techniques can be traced back to the 1950s and 1960s, with foundational studies by researchers such as Dubois, Botnick, and Mead. These pioneering studies sought to explore the mechanical properties of the lungs under different conditions of airflow and pressure.

Impulse oscillometry, as it is used today, was developed more comprehensively in the 1980s and 1990s. Initially, forced oscillation methods were used in research settings to study respiratory mechanics in animals. Over time, advancements in sensor technology, signal processing, and computational models made it possible to adapt this method for human use. Modern IOS technology utilizes high-frequency oscillatory signals that are sent into the respiratory system and then measured to determine the mechanical characteristics of the lungs and airways.

Key Features and Principles of IOS

Impulse oscillometry involves applying small pressure oscillations to the airway at different frequencies and measuring how these oscillations are transmitted through the respiratory system. The response of the respiratory system to these oscillations provides valuable information about lung mechanics, particularly airway resistance and reactance.

Key parameters measured in IOS include:

- *Resistance (R)*: Reflects the opposition to airflow in the airways. Higher resistance typically indicates narrowing or obstruction of the airways.
- *Reactance (X)*: Represents the elasticity or compliance of the airways. Negative reactance values indicate increased stiffness of the airways, often seen in obstructive lung diseases.
- *Resonant frequency*: The frequency at which the airway reactance equals zero and is useful in determining the overall mechanical properties of the lungs.

IOS tests typically involve generating pressure oscillations at frequencies between 5–30 Hz. The resulting data is then analyzed to produce an impedance spectrum, from which resistance and reactance values are extracted.

Importance of IOS in Modern Pulmonary Diagnostics

In clinical practice, IOS has become increasingly recognized for its ability to assess small airway function—something that traditional pulmonary function tests, such as spirometry, often fail to measure effectively. Small airways (those smaller than 2 mm in diameter) play a critical role in overall lung function, and dysfunction in these areas can be a sign of early respiratory disease.

IOS is non-invasive and offers several advantages over traditional methods. Unlike spirometry, which measures airflow during forced exhalation, IOS provides a comprehensive assessment of both the large and small airways, even when the patient cannot perform forced maneuvers. As such, IOS is highly beneficial in diagnosing early-stage airway disease, especially in conditions such as asthma, chronic obstructive pulmonary disease (COPD), and interstitial lung diseases (ILDs).

The non-invasive nature of IOS makes it suitable for repeated measurements, enabling clinicians to monitor disease progression and response to treatment over time without subjecting patients to the discomfort of traditional invasive procedures.

PHYSIOLOGY OF AIRWAYS AND RESPIRATORY SYSTEM

Anatomy and Function of the Respiratory System

The human respiratory system is divided into two primary sections: The conducting zone and the respiratory zone. The conducting zone includes the trachea, bronchi, and bronchioles, which function primarily to transport air to the alveoli. The respiratory zone consists of the alveoli, where gas exchange occurs.

Airway resistance is mainly determined by the caliber of the airways, their length, and the viscosity of the air. In healthy individuals, the majority of airway resistance comes from the larger airways. However, in diseases such as asthma or COPD, smaller airways (which constitute a much smaller percentage of total airway volume) can become critically involved in airflow obstruction.

Airway resistance and lung compliance are essential for maintaining optimal ventilation and gas exchange. Any dysfunction in these properties can lead to impaired respiratory mechanics, which is why accurate measurement of airway resistance is crucial in diagnosing and managing respiratory diseases.

Airway Mechanics and Lung Physiology

Lung compliance refers to the ability of the lungs to expand in response to pressure changes. It is influenced by the elastic properties of lung tissues and the surface tension in the alveoli. Decreased compliance is seen in conditions such as pulmonary fibrosis and acute respiratory distress syndrome (ARDS), where the lungs become stiffer and less able to expand.

Airway resistance, on the other hand, refers to the opposition to airflow within the airways. It is influenced by several factors, including the diameter of the airways, the viscosity of the air, and the airway smooth muscle tone. The resistance is higher in smaller airways, making them particularly susceptible to obstruction in diseases such as asthma and COPD.

Impulse oscillometry measures these resistances and reactances in both large and small airways. By understanding the mechanical properties of the airways and lung tissue, IOS can provide critical insights into the pathophysiology of respiratory diseases.

WHY SMALL AIRWAYS MATTER IN RESPIRATORY MEDICINE?

Small airways are the first to be affected in many common pulmonary diseases. These airways contribute to the total resistance to airflow, and even minor changes in their function can have significant effects on overall lung performance. Diseases such as asthma, COPD, and ILD can cause early changes in the small airways, leading to difficulty in breathing, exercise intolerance, and decreased gas exchange efficiency.

In asthma, for instance, the small airways are often affected by bronchoconstriction and inflammation. Similarly, in COPD, the small airways can undergo remodeling and narrowing due to chronic inflammation and fibrosis. Identifying dysfunction in the small airways early in the disease process is crucial for preventing progression to more severe disease and managing symptoms effectively.

Traditional pulmonary function tests like spirometry are often unable to detect early changes in small airway function. Spirometry measures the flow of air through larger airways during forced exhalation, but small airways contribute relatively little to overall airflow during such tests. This limitation has led to a growing interest in alternative diagnostic methods, such as IOS, which can evaluate both large and small airways.

CURRENT METHODS FOR MEASURING SMALL AIRWAY OBSTRUCTION

Spirometry and Its Limitations in Assessing Small Airways

Spirometry is one of the most commonly used methods for assessing lung function in clinical practice. It measures *forced expiratory volume in 1 second* (FEV_1) and *forced vital capacity (FVC)* during a maximal forced exhalation. These parameters are key indicators of *large airway function* and overall lung volume. However, spirometry is *limited* in assessing the function of small airways. FEF25–75 is often used as a marker of small airway dysfunction, however, it lacks sensitivity and is affected by other parameters.

Small airways—those with a diameter of less than 2 mm—play a significant role in overall airway resistance but are not directly measured by spirometry. In conditions such as *asthma, COPD,* and *bronchitis,* small airways can become *obstructed or narrowed* without affecting the larger airways significantly enough to alter FEV_1 or *FVC* readings. This is especially problematic in early-stage diseases, where changes in *small airway function* can be the *first sign of pathology.*

Furthermore, spirometry requires *maximal effort* from the patient, which may be difficult for children, the elderly, or patients with severe disease. For these reasons, *alternative methods* are necessary to assess small airway dysfunction early and more accurately.

Lung Volume Measurements

Lung volume measurements are conducted using *body plethysmography* or *helium dilution* to assess the total lung capacity (TLC), functional residual capacity (FRC), and residual volume (RV). These measurements help provide insight into the overall condition of the lung and can highlight *hyperinflation* or *air trapping.*

While lung volume measurements can provide indirect clues about small airway function, they are *not specific* to small airway pathology. For example, increased *RV* or *FRC* may suggest *air trapping,* which can be a consequence of *small airway obstruction*; however, these methods do not provide a direct measurement of small airway resistance or reactance, which is where *IOS* excels.

Multiple Breath Nitrogen Washout Test

The *multiple breath nitrogen washout (MBW)* test is another advanced method used to assess small airway function. During the MBW test, a patient inhales a washout gas (typically *100% oxygen*), and the nitrogen concentration is measured as the subject exhales. The test identifies areas of the lung that are poorly ventilated or have impaired gas exchange. This technique is especially useful for detecting *early-stage small airway dysfunction.*

Although the MBW test can provide valuable information about lung ventilation and distribution, it is complex, requires specific equipment, and is not as widely available as *IOS*. Additionally, the MBW test requires *cooperation* from the patient and is more time-consuming, which can limit its practicality in certain settings, especially for pediatric or elderly patients.

Forced Oscillatory Techniques and Impulse Oscillometry

Forced oscillatory techniques (FOT) refer to a class of methods that involve applying a *small oscillating pressure* to the airway to measure the *resistive* and *reactive properties* of the respiratory system. IOS is one of the most prominent methods within FOT. It involves *small pressure waves* of varying frequencies applied to the airways, with the corresponding *response* measured to assess airway resistance and reactance.

The *impulse oscillation* method differs from traditional spirometry in that it can be performed without the need for forced exhalation. This makes it *ideal for young children, elderly patients,* or those with ***severe obstructive diseases*** who may be unable to produce forced exhalations. Moreover, IOS can be used to assess both the *large and small airways,* providing more *detailed information* about airway dysfunction than spirometry or lung volume measurements.

The development of IOS is the result of advancements in *signal processing,* allowing for the use of *high-frequency oscillations* that can measure small airway resistance across a *range of frequencies,* giving detailed insights into the mechanical properties of the entire respiratory system.

THE FORCED OSCILLATION TECHNIQUE AND IMPULSE OSCILLOMETRY

Overview of Forced Oscillation Technique

In *FOT,* the lung impedance is measured across a wide range of frequencies (typically from 5 to 20 Hz). The response to these oscillations is analyzed to differentiate between the effects of *resistance* and *reactance.* Higher frequency oscillations primarily reflect *large airway resistance,* while lower frequency oscillations provide insights into *small airway resistance* and the *elastic properties* of the lungs.

What is Impulse Oscillometry?

Impulse oscillometry is a method within the FOT that specifically uses *short bursts of oscillatory signals* to assess the mechanical properties of the airways. IOS allows for *continuous measurement* of *airway resistance* and *reactance* across various frequencies, providing a *detailed picture* of both large and small airway function.

The process of *IOS* involves sending a short *impulse* into the respiratory system and measuring the response as the signal travels through the airways. This method can measure *resistance* at both high and low frequencies (R5 for high-frequency resistance and R20 for low-frequency resistance), which gives clinicians valuable information about *both central and peripheral airways.*

Technological Advancements in IOS Devices

Over the years, IOS technology has undergone significant advancements. Modern *IOS devices* are compact, portable, and capable of performing real-time measurements with high precision. These devices often use sophisticated *signal processing algorithms* to extract meaningful data from the complex oscillatory signals, enabling precise assessments of *airway resistance* and *reactance* at different frequencies.

The development of *user-friendly interfaces* for IOS devices has made the technique more accessible and practical for routine use in clinical practice. Additionally, improvements in *calibration, accuracy,* and *reproducibility* have enhanced the reliability of IOS as a diagnostic tool for respiratory diseases.

ADVANTAGES OF IMPULSE OSCILLOMETRY OVER TRADITIONAL METHODS

Comparing IOS with Spirometry

Spirometry, while an essential tool for diagnosing and monitoring pulmonary diseases, is *limited* in assessing small airway dysfunction. *Small airways*—those with diameters smaller than 2 mm are responsible for a significant portion of *airway resistance*, but their function is often overlooked in spirometry testing, which primarily assesses large airway function.

In contrast, IOS can assess airway resistance and reactance across both large and small airways. As *small airway disease* is often an early indicator of *chronic respiratory conditions* such as *asthma* and *COPD*, the ability to detect changes in small airway function is crucial for early diagnosis and treatment. Moreover, *IOS is non-invasive, quick*, and requires less patient effort compared to spirometry, making it ideal for use in children, the elderly, and patients with severe respiratory conditions.

IOS and Its Ability to Measure Small Airway Resistance

Impulse oscillometry is particularly valuable because it directly measures *resistance in small airways*, an area traditionally difficult to assess. Unlike spirometry, which requires maximal effort from the patient, *IOS is less affected by patient cooperation* and does not require forced maneuvers. As a result, IOS can detect *small airway dysfunction* in the *early stages of disease*, often before more overt symptoms such as *dyspnea* (shortness of breath) or *wheezing* appear.

By using multiple frequencies, IOS can assess *frequency-dependent resistance*, enabling clinicians to identify changes in *airway reactance* and *resistance* that might otherwise go undetected. This level of detail makes IOS a highly sensitive and reliable tool for diagnosing and monitoring diseases such as *asthma, COPD*, and *pulmonary fibrosis*.

HOW TO PERFORM IMPULSE OSCILLOMETRY?

Patient Preparation for IOS Testing

IOS is a relatively straightforward test to perform and requires minimal patient preparation. However, to ensure accurate and reliable results, there are a few considerations to keep in mind:

- *Pre-test instructions*: Patients should avoid consuming food or drinks that could increase airway resistance, such as caffeine or alcohol, for several hours before the test. It is also advisable to avoid using bronchodilators before the test unless otherwise instructed by a healthcare provider.
- *Equipment calibration*: IOS devices must be calibrated according to the manufacturer's instructions before use. Regular calibration is essential to ensure the accuracy of the results.
- *Positioning*: The patient should be seated comfortably in an upright position to allow optimal airway function during testing. A proper *nose clip* may be used to prevent airflow through the nostrils and ensure that the patient is breathing through their mouth.

- *Breathing instructions*: Patients should be instructed to breathe *normally* through the mouthpiece during the test, which typically takes only a few minutes. It is crucial that the patient remains *relaxed* and *comfortable* to avoid any unnecessary stress that could impact the results.

Step-by-step Procedure for IOS Measurements

- *Patient calibration*: Before the actual test begins, the device is calibrated, and the patient's respiratory impedance is measured at baseline. This step ensures that the device is working properly.
- *Oscillatory signal application*: The test begins by applying a series of oscillatory signals at varying frequencies. The patient continues to breathe normally while the device measures how the oscillations are transmitted through the airways.
- *Data collection*: As the patient breathes normally, the device collects data on both airway resistance and reactance. This data is then processed using sophisticated algorithms to generate a detailed impedance spectrum.
- *Test duration*: The entire test typically takes about 5–10 minutes, with only a few minutes of actual oscillatory signal exposure. The test is non-invasive and generally well-tolerated by patients.
- *Post-test evaluation*: After the test, the clinician evaluates the results, which include airway resistance (R) and reactance (X) at different frequencies. The data can be compared to normative values and used to identify any abnormalities.

WHEN TO PERFORM IMPULSE OSCILLOMETRY?

Indications for IOS in Clinical Practice

Impulse oscillometry has become an essential tool for assessing lung function, especially in diseases where *small airway dysfunction* is a key feature. While traditional methods like spirometry are commonly used for diagnosing obstructive lung diseases, IOS offers more nuanced and sensitive measurements of *airway resistance* and *reactance*, particularly in the *small airways*.

Some specific indications for performing IOS include:

- *Early detection of obstructive lung diseases*: IOS can identify changes in airway function before spirometry reveals any abnormal results. In conditions such as *asthma* or *COPD*, where small airway involvement is common, IOS can detect *small airway obstruction* even in the early stages of disease. This is critical for initiating early intervention before irreversible damage occurs.
- *Evaluation of asthma*: Asthma is characterized by *bronchoconstriction* and *airway hyperreactivity*, which often involves the small airways. IOS can help assess the degree of obstruction and monitor response to *bronchodilators* or *steroid therapy*. It can also be used to track *bronchial responsiveness* over time, making it valuable for disease management and progression.
- *Assessment of COPD*: In *COPD*, the progressive narrowing of the airways leads to *airflow limitation*, especially in the small airways. IOS can help assess *small airway function* early in the disease course, even before changes in FEV_1

become noticeable. Regular monitoring with IOS can guide the management of *COPD* and help assess the effectiveness of treatment strategies.

- *Children and infants*: IOS has a significant advantage over spirometry in pediatric populations, especially in younger children and infants who may not be able to perform forced expiratory maneuvers. IOS testing requires *minimal cooperation*, and the procedure is quick and non-invasive. It is particularly useful in *diagnosing asthma* and *tracking airway resistance* in children with respiratory symptoms.
- *Monitoring airway disease progression*: IOS can be used to monitor the progression of diseases such as *bronchiectasis*, *cystic fibrosis*, and *pulmonary fibrosis*, where small airway involvement plays a key role in disease development. Regular monitoring with IOS allows clinicians to evaluate changes in *airway function* and *lung mechanics*, helping to assess disease severity and response to treatment.
- *Evaluation of response to therapy*: One of the key advantages of IOS is its ability to assess the *immediate response* to bronchodilators, corticosteroids, or other therapeutic interventions. For example, a reduction in *airway resistance* after a bronchodilator administration is a key indicator of effective therapy. IOS can be used to evaluate bronchodilator reversibility, providing real-time feedback on the effectiveness of treatment regimens.
- *Preoperative assessment*: In patients undergoing *thoracic surgery* or *lung transplantation*, IOS can be used to evaluate *preoperative airway function*. Since small airway dysfunction can influence postoperative recovery, measuring small airway resistance can provide useful information to guide *perioperative care*.
- *Assessment of respiratory conditions with limited spirometry utility*: In patients who are unable to perform traditional spirometry, such as those with *neuromuscular diseases*, *severe COPD*, or *pediatric patients*, IOS can be a valuable alternative. It does not require forced exhalation or patient effort, making it more accessible for these populations.

HOW TO INTERPRET RESULTS FROM IMPULSE OSCILLOMETRY?

Key Parameters Measured in IOS

To interpret IOS results effectively, it is crucial to understand the various parameters generated during the test. These parameters provide insights into the *mechanical properties* of the respiratory system. The main parameters that are typically analyzed in IOS are:

- *Airway resistance (R) at multiple frequencies*:
    - R5 (high-frequency resistance): Represents resistance in the large airways.
    - R20 (low-frequency resistance): Reflects the overall resistance across the entire respiratory system, including the small airways.
    - R10, R15: Intermediate frequencies that can give more detailed information about both the large and small airways.

- *Airway reactance (X)*: Reactance refers to the elastic properties of the airways, such as *compliance* (ability to expand and contract). Negative values of reactance typically indicate airway constriction or increased *stiffness* in the lungs. Reactance is measured at low frequencies (e.g., X5, X10) and provides information about *small airway compliance.*
- *Resonance frequency (fres)*: Resonance frequency is the frequency at which the respiratory system exhibits the maximum response to oscillatory forces. The *fres* can be used to assess overall lung compliance and help in identifying abnormal lung mechanics.

Interpreting Increased Resistance

When resistance measurements, particularly *R5* and *R20,* are elevated, it suggests that there is *obstruction* or *narrowing* of the airways. An increase in *R20* is typically seen in patients with *obstructive pulmonary diseases* such as *asthma* or *COPD,* where inflammation and bronchoconstriction lead to increased airway resistance. *Elevated R5* indicates that the *larger airways* are also affected, but *increased R20* is a more specific indicator of *small airway dysfunction.*

The key to interpretation lies in understanding the *frequency dependence* of resistance. In cases of *small airway obstruction,* resistance often increases disproportionately at *lower frequencies* (e.g., R5 > R20), indicating *more pronounced changes in the smaller airways* compared to the larger ones.

Using Prime Numbers for Impulse Oscillometry Interpretation

Using prime numbers is based on the principle that resistance measurements taken at odd-numbered frequencies provide better resolution in detecting changes in *small airway resistance.* R20 may be sensitive to harmonic variability. As such, *R19* is considered to be a more accurate representation of *peripheral airway resistance,* allowing for more precise diagnostic interpretation.

Interpretation of Reactance (X) Values

Reactance provides insight into the *elastic properties* of the airways. A *negative reactance* value (i.e., when X < 0) is indicative of increased *airway stiffness,* which may be due to *airway remodeling, fibrosis,* or *inflammation* in diseases such as *asthma, COPD,* or *pulmonary fibrosis.*

Changes in *reactance* can also be used to evaluate *bronchodilator response.* A reduction in *reactance* following bronchodilator administration suggests a positive response to the medication, as the airways become less stiff and more compliant.

Bronchodilator Reversibility Criteria

IOS is a valuable tool for assessing bronchodilator reversibility, particularly in conditions like asthma. It is more sensitive than spirometry in detecting changes in small airways.

Criteria for Bronchodilator Response

- *Resistance (R)*:
  - A decrease in R_5 of ≥40% from baseline indicates significant improvement in total airway resistance.
  - A reduction in R_5 - R_{20} of ≥50% suggests significant improvement in small airway function.
  - In the odd numbers method, a similar threshold applies to R_5 - R_{19}.
- *Reactance (X)*:
  - An increase in X_5 (i.e., less negative) of ≥50% from baseline suggests improved compliance and reduced small airway obstruction.
  - A significant reduction in AX (≥50%) indicates decreased hyperinflation and improved distal airway function.

Advantages of IOS in Bronchodilator Testing

- *Small airway sensitivity*: IOS can detect small airway improvement even when spirometric changes (e.g., FEV_1) are minimal.
- *Effort-independent testing*: Particularly useful in patients who struggle to perform forced maneuvers required in spirometry.

Introduction to Intra-breath Oscillometry

Intra-breath oscillometry (IBO) is an advanced modification of traditional IOS that allows for the continuous measurement of respiratory mechanics during a natural tidal breathing cycle. Unlike conventional IOS, which measures airway resistance and reactance during forced breathing maneuvers, *IBO* integrates respiratory impedance measurements within the *breathing cycle* itself, enabling more dynamic and real-time data collection during normal, unforced *tidal breathing*. This method enhances the ability to assess airway function under more physiological conditions, making it particularly valuable in both clinical and research settings where forced maneuvers may be difficult to obtain or less representative of everyday lung function.

The key feature of IBO is its ability to measure *airway resistance, reactance,* and other respiratory parameters during different phases of the breathing cycle, providing more granular insights into the *temporal variability* of airway function. This can be crucial for understanding *small airway dynamics, airway responsiveness,* and *ventilation distribution* in a more representative, non-invasive manner.

Technical Principles of Intra-breath Oscillometry

Intra-breath oscillometry builds upon the principles of standard IOS but operates with some key modifications. In both IOS and IBO, oscillations are generated and delivered into the airways, but the main difference lies in the timing and how the signals are recorded.

- *Oscillatory signal generation*: In IBO, a set of *high-frequency pressure oscillations* (typically ranging from 5 to 35 Hz) is introduced into the airways during the *inspiratory* and *expiratory phases* of the *tidal breathing cycle.* These oscillations are delivered continuously, allowing for measurement of respiratory impedance throughout the breath. This contrasts with traditional IOS, where oscillations are applied only during forced exhalation, typically at a constant frequency.

- *Measurement of respiratory impedance*: IBO measures *airway resistance* (R), *reactance* (X), and *impedance* (Z) continuously throughout the breathing cycle. The impedance can be analyzed at various frequencies, with the most significant values typically being at the low-frequency end (representing large airway contributions) and high-frequency end (reflecting small airway function). The primary goal of IBO is to capture real-time changes in *airway mechanics* during *natural breathing* and assess how these change from one breath to another.
- *Phase-specific measurements*: A significant advantage of IBO is its ability to measure changes in *airway mechanics* across different phases of a single breath (i.e., during *inspiration, expiration,* and *breath holding*). This provides a more detailed picture of how the airways behave under normal physiological conditions. For example, by analyzing *impedance* during the expiratory phase, clinicians can identify any changes or resistance caused by *airway narrowing, bronchoconstriction,* or *increased airway viscosity,* which might not be evident during forced maneuvers

CLINICAL APPLICATIONS OF IMPULSE OSCILLOMETRY

Impulse oscillometry has proven to be a valuable tool in clinical settings, offering more precise and comprehensive insights into airway mechanics than traditional methods. The clinical applications of IOS extend across a wide range of respiratory conditions, including asthma, COPD, pulmonary fibrosis, and more.

Asthma Management

IOS is particularly useful in *asthma management,* where small airway obstruction plays a key role. Asthma exacerbations are often caused by *bronchoconstriction,* which affects the *small airways.* By regularly assessing *airway resistance* and *reactance,* clinicians can detect *early signs of airway narrowing* and track the effectiveness of *bronchodilator therapy.* IOS also helps identify patients who might benefit from *inhaled corticosteroids* or *long-acting beta agonists.*

Chronic Obstructive Pulmonary Disease

Impulse oscillometry has become a valuable diagnostic tool for assessing *small airway dysfunction* in *COPD.* While traditional methods such as spirometry typically focus on large airway function, IOS enables clinicians to detect abnormalities in the *small airways* early on, even before spirometry shows a reduction in FEV_1.

- *Detecting small airway involvement*: In *COPD*, small airway dysfunction is thought to play a crucial role in disease progression. Changes in the *R5* and *R20* parameters measured by IOS reflect *airway resistance* in both the small and large airways, making it easier to assess the *severity of small airway involvement*. The detection of increased *frequency dependence of resistance*, characterized by a higher *R5/R20* ratio, is often an early sign of *airway remodeling* and *obstruction* in COPD.
- *Monitoring disease progression*: IOS can help track the progression of *COPD* by measuring subtle changes in *airway resistance* and *reactance* over time. Since small airway dysfunction can precede large airway changes, IOS allows clinicians to assess early functional decline, even before overt symptoms or spirometric changes occur. It can also be used to monitor the response to interventions such as *bronchodilators*, *corticosteroids*, or *pulmonary rehabilitation*.
- *Assessing bronchodilator response*: One of the most important applications of IOS in COPD is its ability to assess *bronchodilator reversibility*. After administering a bronchodilator, IOS can measure how the airway resistance and reactance change in response. In *COPD*, bronchodilator responses tend to be less pronounced than in asthma, but significant improvements in *R5* or *R20* following treatment may indicate a *reversible component* of the disease. This information can help tailor treatment plans and determine the effectiveness of bronchodilators.
- *Evaluating impact of therapy*: IOS can be used to assess the effectiveness of various treatments, including *inhaled bronchodilators*, *steroids*, and *anticholinergic agents*. In patients with *moderate-to-severe COPD*, where airway remodeling may lead to irreversible changes, IOS can provide valuable information on the degree of *small airway involvement* that might still be reversible with pharmacological interventions.

Pulmonary Fibrosis and Interstitial Lung Diseases

Pulmonary fibrosis and other *ILDs* often involve changes in the *small airways*, leading to *restrictive patterns* and *reduced gas exchange*. While *spirometry* may indicate a reduction in *lung volumes*, it does not provide a complete picture of *small airway function*. IOS, by assessing both *airway resistance* and *reactance*, provides additional insights into the condition of the *small airways* in patients with ILD.

- *Detecting early changes*: In *pulmonary fibrosis*, early changes in *airway resistance* and *reactance* often occur before changes in **spirometry**. IOS can detect early *small airway dysfunction*, even in the absence of overt *airflow limitation* or *restrictive patterns* in conventional tests. Increased *frequency dependence of resistance* is often observed in *ILDs*, indicating early alterations in small airway function.
- *Monitoring disease progression*: Since *pulmonary fibrosis* and other ILDs involve ongoing *fibrosis* and *scarring* of the lung tissue, monitoring small airway function with IOS can help assess the *progression* of the disease. Increased airway resistance and reactance values over time can signal

worsening disease, providing early indicators of worsening *lung function*. This allows for timely interventions to prevent further decline.

Children and Infants

One of the most significant advantages of IOS is its ability to evaluate lung function in populations where traditional pulmonary function tests, such as spirometry, are difficult to perform. *Children*, particularly *infants and toddlers*, may not be able to perform forced expiratory maneuvers, making conventional tests unsuitable. IOS, however, requires minimal cooperation and can provide valuable data on *airway resistance* and *reactance*.

- *Diagnosing asthma in children*: Asthma is the most common chronic respiratory disease in children. IOS provides an effective means of diagnosing asthma in younger patients who may have difficulty completing spirometry. Increased *R5* and *R20* values are indicative of *bronchoconstriction* in asthma. Tracking these values over time can also help assess treatment efficacy and adjust asthma management strategies.
- *Assessing airway function in infants*: In infants, especially those under the age of two, performing spirometry can be technically challenging or even impossible. IOS, however, can be conducted in infants as young as *6 months old*, making it an ideal tool for assessing early airway resistance and tracking the progress of diseases such as asthma, *bronchiolitis*, or *cystic fibrosis*.
- *Monitoring response to treatment*: In pediatric patients, especially those with *asthma*, IOS can help monitor how the airways respond to treatment. Following bronchodilator administration, a reduction in *airway resistance* is expected, and IOS provides real-time feedback on whether the airways are responding appropriately. This helps guide therapeutic decisions and ensures that children receive the most effective interventions for their condition.

FUTURE DIRECTIONS AND INNOVATIONS IN IMPULSE OSCILLOMETRY

Impulse oscillometry has undergone significant advancements over the past few decades, and ongoing research is expanding the potential applications of this technique. As technology improves, IOS may play an even greater role in clinical practice, offering more sensitive, specific, and accessible methods for assessing *small airway dysfunction* and *lung mechanics*.

Development of More Advanced Algorithms

As data collection and analysis techniques improve, more advanced algorithms could be developed to analyze IOS measurements. For example, incorporating machine learning and *artificial intelligence (AI)* could enable more accurate prediction of disease progression, response to treatment, and even early diagnosis of conditions such as *COPD* or *asthma*. These algorithms could help clinicians make *better-informed decisions* based on patient-specific data, improving both diagnostics and treatment outcomes.

CHAPTER 4

Diffusing Capacity of the Lung for Carbon Monoxide

INTRODUCTION TO DLCO

The Role of DLCO in Pulmonary Medicine

The diffusing capacity of the lung for carbon monoxide (DLCO) is an essential diagnostic tool in modern respiratory medicine, offering profound insight into the ability of the lungs to transfer gases from the alveoli to the blood. Unlike traditional spirometry that assesses airflow, DLCO specifically evaluates the efficiency of gas exchange across the alveolar-capillary barrier. By measuring the diffusion of carbon monoxide (CO), a gas with high affinity for hemoglobin, DLCO testing provides a sensitive measure of the overall functional status of the lungs, which is crucial in understanding various pulmonary conditions.

The Importance of DLCO

The clinical utility of DLCO lies in its ability to detect subtle changes in lung function that other tests might miss, especially in the early stages of diseases that impair gas exchange. These include interstitial lung diseases (ILDs), chronic obstructive pulmonary disease (COPD), pulmonary hypertension, and conditions like pulmonary fibrosis. DLCO testing is indispensable for:

- *Identifying the severity and progression of ILD*, where fibrosis thickens the alveolar-capillary membrane and reduces gas transfer.
- *Diagnosing obstructive lung diseases* like emphysema, where loss of alveolar surface area results in decreased gas exchange.
- *Monitoring the effects of treatments*, including the use of bronchodilators in patients with asthma and the evaluation of pulmonary vascular diseases like pulmonary hypertension.
- *Assessing preoperative lung function*, particularly in lung resection surgery or lung transplantation, to predict postoperative outcomes.

Historical Development of DLCO Testing

The use of DLCO testing dates back to the early 20th century, when researchers sought a method to assess the efficiency of gas exchange. Early studies in respiratory physiology introduced CO as an ideal tracer due to its high affinity for hemoglobin, which allowed researchers to measure how well the lungs could transfer gases across the alveolar-capillary barrier. The development of the single-breath method of DLCO measurement in the 1950s marked a significant leap forward, and since then, improvements in testing techniques and standardization of protocols have made DLCO one of the most reliable measures of pulmonary function.

THE PHYSIOLOGY OF GAS EXCHANGE IN THE LUNGS

The Alveolar-capillary Membrane

Gas exchange in the lungs takes place across the alveolar-capillary membrane, which consists of several layers: The alveolar epithelium, the interstitial space, the capillary endothelium, and the red blood cells. The membrane must be thin, but large enough to provide sufficient surface area for gas exchange to meet the body's needs. The efficiency of this exchange depends on several factors:

- *Surface area of the alveolar membrane*: The larger the surface area, the more gas can be exchanged. Diseases such as emphysema cause the destruction of alveolar walls, reducing surface area and thereby decreasing diffusion capacity.
- *Thickness of the alveolar-capillary membrane*: A thinner membrane allows for more efficient gas transfer. In contrast, conditions like pulmonary fibrosis thicken the membrane, leading to impaired diffusion.
- *Perfusion and ventilation balance*: Adequate blood flow is necessary to transport oxygen from the alveoli to the tissues. A mismatch in ventilation and perfusion, seen in conditions like pulmonary embolism or pulmonary hypertension, can reduce diffusion capacity.
- *Hemoglobin concentration*: Hemoglobin carries oxygen in the blood. The ability of the blood to carry CO, which competes for hemoglobin binding sites, directly affects DLCO readings.

Diffusion of Gases: The Key Factors

Diffusion, the process by which gases move from areas of high concentration to areas of low concentration, is governed by Fick's Law, which states that the rate of diffusion is proportional to the surface area and the partial pressure gradient of the gas, and inversely proportional to the thickness of the membrane. The diffusion of CO in the lungs follows this principle, with CO acting as a proxy for oxygen due to its similar molecular weight and diffusivity but significantly higher affinity for hemoglobin.

In healthy individuals, oxygen diffusion in the lungs is rapid and efficient due to an optimal surface area, minimal membrane thickness, and robust blood flow. Any disease that alters these factors can reduce DLCO and impair gas exchange, making DLCO testing a critical tool in diagnosing and monitoring these conditions.

Why Carbon Monoxide is Preferable for Measuring DLCO?

High Affinity for Hemoglobin

One of the primary reasons CO is chosen over other gases is its **extremely high** *affinity for hemoglobin.* CO binds to hemoglobin about 200–250 times more strongly than oxygen. This property makes it an ideal gas for measuring the capacity of the lungs to transfer gases to the bloodstream. When CO is inhaled during DLCO testing, it readily binds to hemoglobin in the red blood cells, mimicking the behavior of oxygen, but in a more controlled and measurable way.

This high affinity is crucial for the *sensitivity and specificity* of DLCO measurements. Since CO is quickly absorbed into the bloodstream upon inhalation, the amount of CO that remains in the alveolar space can be directly correlated with the amount of CO that has diffused across the alveolar-capillary barrier, allowing for accurate measurement of diffusion capacity.

Minimal Competing Reactions

Unlike oxygen or other gases, *CO undergoes very few competing reactions in the lungs and bloodstream.* For instance, oxygen is used by cells for cellular respiration, while CO, once bound to hemoglobin, remains in the bloodstream for the duration of the test, without being consumed or metabolized. This makes CO particularly effective for DLCO measurements because its fate can be easily tracked, and its diffusion through the alveolar-capillary membrane can be accurately quantified.

Furthermore, the *minimal metabolic activity* of CO allows for a stable and consistent measurement. This is in contrast to gases like oxygen or nitrogen, which undergo various physiological processes such as oxygen utilization in tissues, reducing the reliability of diffusion measurements over time.

Low Background Concentrations in the Body

Another key reason CO is used in DLCO testing is that it is *naturally present in very low concentrations in the human body.* While trace amounts of CO can be produced in the body during cellular respiration and other metabolic processes, these levels are negligible and do not interfere with DLCO measurements. This contrasts with gases like oxygen or carbon dioxide, which are present in significant amounts in the lungs and bloodstream and would require complex calculations to account for their levels.

The low natural concentration of CO in the body means that its measurement during DLCO testing reflects primarily the diffusion process, without interference from other physiological factors. This results in more accurate and reproducible measurements of diffusion capacity.

Easy Detection and Measurement

Carbon monoxide is *easy to detect and measure,* which is another important reason it is used in DLCO testing. The gas has a strong absorbance in the infrared spectrum, which allows for precise measurement even at low concentrations. Modern DLCO analyzers are equipped with highly sensitive detectors that can measure CO concentrations with a high degree of accuracy.

Other gases, such as oxygen or nitrous oxide, would be more difficult to measure with the same level of precision due to their lower detectability and the need for more complex equipment to monitor their concentrations in the exhaled breath.

Mimicking Oxygen Diffusion

Carbon monoxide is chemically similar to oxygen in terms of its ability to diffuse across the alveolar-capillary membrane. Both gases are small, nonpolar molecules that can diffuse passively down a concentration gradient. However, CO has a higher affinity for hemoglobin, which allows it to *serve as a surrogate for oxygen* in the measurement of lung diffusion capacity.

The diffusion of CO in the lungs is essentially a *proxy for the diffusion of oxygen*, as both gases behave similarly in the lungs, but CO provides a more controlled and quantifiable means to assess the efficiency of gas exchange. The use of CO in DLCO testing, therefore, allows for an accurate estimate of how efficiently the lungs are able to transfer oxygen to the bloodstream, which is crucial for assessing lung function in various pulmonary diseases.

Safety Profile of Carbon Monoxide in Controlled Doses

Despite its toxic properties at high concentrations, *CO is safe for use in very low, controlled doses* during DLCO testing. The amount of CO used in a typical DLCO test is well below harmful levels and does not pose a risk to the patient. The typical concentration of CO used in the test is about 0.1% (1,000 ppm), and the exposure time is brief—lasting only a few seconds during the breath-holding phase. This makes the test both *safe and effective.*

Moreover, the body has mechanisms for removing small amounts of CO from the bloodstream. Once the test is complete and the patient exhales, the CO is quickly eliminated from the body through the lungs, and the levels return to baseline within a short period.

Accurate Measurement of Diffusion Capacity

The most critical reason for using CO in DLCO testing is that it *provides an accurate measurement of the lungs' diffusion capacity.* The diffusion of CO through the alveolar-capillary membrane is directly related to the surface area available for gas exchange, the thickness of the membrane, and the ability of the blood to absorb the gas. By measuring how much CO is absorbed and how much remains in the alveolar space, clinicians can assess the efficiency of the lungs in transferring gases.

Other gases, such as oxygen or nitrogen, are not as effective at providing this kind of information due to their different behaviors in the bloodstream and lungs. For example, nitrogen is inert and does not bind to hemoglobin, which would make it a less useful measure of diffusion capacity, as it would not reflect the lung's ability to transfer gases into the blood.

Stability and Consistency of Results

The use of CO provides *consistent and reliable results* over time. Because the gas is not metabolized and does not participate in cellular processes, its concentration in the alveoli and bloodstream remains stable during the breath-hold phase. This allows for more reproducible and accurate measurements compared to other gases, which may show variations due to metabolic consumption or other factors.

Additionally, the diffusion of CO is less influenced by external variables such as exercise or ambient conditions, which may affect the diffusion of gases like oxygen or carbon dioxide. This stability makes CO an ideal choice for *standardized clinical testing*, ensuring that results can be reliably compared across different patients and different testing environments.

CLINICAL APPLICATIONS OF DLCO

Diagnosing Interstitial Lung Diseases

Interstitial lung diseases, a group of over 200 different disorders, affect the interstitial tissues of the lungs, leading to progressive scarring (fibrosis) of lung tissue. This fibrosis thickens the alveolar-capillary membrane, reducing the efficiency of gas exchange and, consequently, the DLCO. Early stages of ILD may not show significant changes in spirometry, but DLCO may be reduced, allowing for earlier detection of the disease. Common ILDs include:

- *Idiopathic pulmonary fibrosis (IPF)*: Characterized by progressive scarring of lung tissue, IPF often leads to a significant reduction in DLCO.
- *Sarcoidosis*: A granulomatous disease that can affect multiple organs, sarcoidosis often leads to decreased DLCO due to granuloma formation in the lung tissue.
- *Systemic sclerosis (scleroderma)*: This autoimmune disease can lead to both pulmonary fibrosis and pulmonary vascular disease, both of which may reduce DLCO.

Chronic Obstructive Pulmonary Disease

Chronic obstructive pulmonary disease is primarily characterized by airflow limitation due to chronic inflammation and narrowing of the airways. Emphysema, one of the key components of COPD, causes the destruction of alveolar walls and a reduction in surface area for gas exchange, leading to a decrease in DLCO. Unlike spirometry, which focuses on airflow limitations, DLCO provides a measure of how well the lungs are able to exchange gases, even in the absence of significant airflow obstruction.

Pulmonary Hypertension and Vascular Disease

Pulmonary hypertension involves elevated pressures in the pulmonary arteries, which can impair blood flow to the lungs and reduce the ability of the lungs to exchange gases. This leads to a reduction in DLCO, and DLCO testing is used to assess the severity of pulmonary vascular diseases and to monitor treatment response.

Preoperative Lung Function Assessment

In patients undergoing lung resection or lung transplantation, DLCO testing is used to assess the remaining functional lung capacity. A reduced DLCO is an indicator of poor lung function and may suggest increased risk of postoperative complications such as respiratory failure or prolonged recovery. DLCO is also used in assessing candidates for lung volume reduction surgery (LVRS) in emphysema.

METHODS OF MEASURING DLCO

The Single-breath DLCO Test

The single-breath method is the most widely used and standardized technique for measuring DLCO. In this test, the patient inhales a gas mixture containing CO and a tracer gas (typically helium or methane), holds their breath for 10 seconds, and then exhales. The exhaled air is analyzed to measure the amount of CO absorbed into the blood during the breath-hold. The test is performed in a series of steps:

- *Preparation*: The patient is instructed to fully exhale to residual volume and then inhale the test gas mixture to total lung capacity.
- *Breath hold*: The patient holds their breath for 10 seconds, during which the CO in the inhaled mixture diffuses into the blood across the alveolar-capillary membrane.
- *Exhalation and analysis*: The patient then exhales into a collection device, and the concentration of CO in the exhaled air is measured.
- *Calculation*: DLCO is calculated based on the amount of CO absorbed, adjusting for factors such as lung volume (using the alveolar volume, VA).

The Steady-state DLCO Method

The steady-state method is less commonly used but can be an alternative for certain patient populations, such as those unable to perform the single-breath maneuver. In this test, the patient breathes in a mixture of CO and tracer gas continuously, and the amount of CO absorbed is measured over time. While less precise than the single-breath method, the steady-state method can be used for patients who cannot hold their breath.

INTERPRETATION OF DLCO RESULTS

Normal DLCO Values

Normal DLCO values vary depending on age, gender, height, weight, and other individual factors. Reference values for DLCO are derived from large population studies and are adjusted for these variables. In healthy adults, the typical DLCO value is approximately 25 mL/min/mm Hg, but it can vary widely. A reduction in DLCO below 80% of the predicted value indicates a decrease in lung diffusion capacity, and values below 60% are considered significantly reduced.

Factors Affecting DLCO Interpretation

- *Hemoglobin levels*: Anemia can artificially lower DLCO, as there is less hemoglobin available to bind CO. Conversely, polycythemia can elevate DLCO.
- *Age and gender*: DLCO naturally declines with age and is generally lower in females.
- *Body size*: Taller individuals typically have higher DLCO values, as they have larger lung volumes and greater alveolar surface area.
- *Smoking*: Smoking may affect DLCO by causing structural changes in the lungs that impair gas exchange, leading to a reduction in DLCO over time.
- *Posture*: DLCO values are generally higher when the patient is in the supine position due to better perfusion of the lungs.

Bronchodilator Reversibility and DLCO

DLCO can also be measured before and after the administration of a bronchodilator to assess reversibility in patients with asthma or COPD. A significant increase in DLCO after bronchodilator use suggests that airway obstruction is reversible, and the improvement in diffusion may reflect improved pulmonary blood flow and reduced ventilation-perfusion mismatch.

DLCO IN SPECIAL POPULATIONS

Pediatric Population

In children, DLCO testing is more challenging due to difficulties in patient cooperation. However, it is invaluable in diagnosing and monitoring conditions such as cystic fibrosis, bronchopulmonary dysplasia, and ILD. Reference values for DLCO in children are adjusted for body size and age, and DLCO is measured using modified techniques, such as the steady-state method, in younger patients.

Geriatric Population

In the elderly, the interpretation of DLCO results must be carefully considered in light of age-related changes in pulmonary function. As people age, there are several physiologic changes that may lead to a decline in DLCO:

- *Decreased alveolar surface area*: With aging, the alveolar walls may become less compliant, leading to reduced surface area available for gas exchange. This results in reduced efficiency in diffusing gases, including CO, across the alveolar-capillary membrane.
- *Reduced pulmonary capillary blood volume*: Aging is also associated with a reduction in the pulmonary capillary network. This reduces the volume of blood available for gas exchange, which may further contribute to a decline in DLCO.
- *Changes in lung compliance*: Older individuals often experience decreased lung compliance, leading to increased resistance to airflow and less efficient ventilation. This can contribute to a decline in DLCO readings.

Additionally, comorbidities that are common in geriatric populations, such as heart failure, pulmonary hypertension, and COPD, can further complicate the interpretation of DLCO results. For instance, pulmonary hypertension and left heart failure may decrease DLCO, even in the absence of significant changes in pulmonary parenchymal structure. Conversely, anemia, which is common in elderly patients, can artificially reduce DLCO by decreasing the hemoglobin concentration in blood, reducing the capacity for CO binding.

Pregnancy

In pregnant women, DLCO may show increased values, particularly in the second and third trimesters. This is largely due to:

- *Increased blood volume*: Pregnancy increases the overall blood volume, which in turn increases the pulmonary capillary blood volume (Vc), enhancing the ability of the lungs to take up gases.
- *Hormonal changes*: Progesterone and other hormones produced during pregnancy can lead to increased ventilation, which in turn affects the diffusion capacity. This is a physiological adaptation to meet the increased oxygen demands during pregnancy.

It's important to note that while DLCO generally increases during pregnancy, pathologic conditions such as preeclampsia, pulmonary embolism, or asthma exacerbations may cause abnormal DLCO values. Therefore, clinical context is crucial when interpreting results in pregnant patients.

DLCO IN DIFFERENT PULMONARY DISEASES

Interstitial Lung Disease

Interstitial lung disease encompasses a wide range of diseases that affect the interstitial spaces of the lungs, leading to inflammation, fibrosis, or granuloma formation. These conditions typically lead to a reduced DLCO due to thickening of the alveolar-capillary membrane, which impairs the diffusion of gases. Some common ILDs include:

- *Idiopathic pulmonary fibrosis*: This chronic, progressive disease is characterized by fibrotic changes in the lung parenchyma, which reduce the surface area available for gas exchange. As the fibrosis progresses, DLCO continues to decrease, making it a critical parameter for monitoring disease progression.
- *Systemic sclerosis (scleroderma)*: Systemic sclerosis can affect both the pulmonary vasculature and the lung parenchyma, resulting in both a reduction in DLCO and impaired lung compliance. Patients with scleroderma-related ILD often exhibit a decreased DLCO before other symptoms appear, which can serve as an early diagnostic indicator.
- *Sarcoidosis*: Sarcoidosis is another disease that may involve the lungs and lead to granulomatous inflammation, which can impair gas diffusion. The presence of granulomas within the interstitial space can cause a decrease in DLCO, although this may not always correlate with pulmonary function testing (PFT) results.

- *Asbestosis and occupational lung diseases*: These diseases, caused by inhalation of toxic particles like asbestos, lead to progressive pulmonary fibrosis and a reduction in DLCO. Often, these diseases are diagnosed later in life, and DLCO can provide useful information for both diagnosis and prognosis.

DLCO is particularly useful for detecting the severity of ILD and monitoring its progression, as changes in DLCO precede changes in spirometry in many ILDs. Additionally, because DLCO is also sensitive to pulmonary vascular disease, it can assist in distinguishing between restrictive lung disease due to parenchymal changes and that due to pulmonary vascular changes.

Chronic Obstructive Pulmonary Disease

Chronic obstructive pulmonary disease is primarily characterized by airflow obstruction resulting from chronic bronchitis and emphysema. Emphysema, in particular, leads to the destruction of alveolar walls and a significant reduction in the surface area for gas exchange. This results in a decreased DLCO, which is often seen in patients with advanced emphysema. However, the degree of DLCO reduction in COPD can vary based on the extent of emphysema and the presence of other comorbidities like pulmonary hypertension.

In patients with COPD, DLCO can be measured both at rest and after the administration of bronchodilators to assess reversibility of airflow obstruction. A non-reversible reduction in DLCO suggests a fixed reduction in alveolar surface area or pulmonary capillary blood volume, which is commonly seen in emphysema. However, in chronic bronchitis, DLCO may not be as markedly reduced, because the primary pathology is airway inflammation rather than alveolar damage.

Pulmonary Vascular Diseases

Pulmonary vascular diseases, such as pulmonary hypertension and pulmonary embolism, can significantly affect DLCO measurements. In pulmonary hypertension, there is increased resistance in the pulmonary vasculature, which leads to impaired blood flow through the lungs and reduced gas exchange. This results in a lowered DLCO. However, the relationship between pulmonary hypertension and DLCO is complex, as early stages of the disease may not lead to a significant decrease in DLCO.

Asthma

In asthma, airway inflammation and bronchoconstriction result in airflow obstruction. However, asthma does not typically affect the alveolar-capillary membrane directly, so DLCO may remain normal or only mildly reduced in stable asthma. During acute exacerbations, DLCO may temporarily improve due to increased pulmonary blood flow, which is a compensatory response to reduced ventilation.

Bronchodilator reversibility testing can help assess the improvement in both spirometry and DLCO after treatment, providing additional diagnostic and prognostic information. In cases where asthma is associated with other comorbidities, such as emphysema, DLCO may be reduced.

Pulmonary Embolism

Pulmonary embolism, a blockage in one of the pulmonary arteries typically caused by a blood clot, can result in decreased perfusion of the lungs. This can impair the diffusion of gases, leading to a reduction in DLCO. DLCO measurement is useful for evaluating the extent of impairment in gas exchange in patients with suspected or confirmed PE. Additionally, PE may lead to ventilation-perfusion mismatching, which can result in an increased alveolar-arterial gradient and abnormal DLCO values.

TECHNIQUES FOR MEASURING DLCO

Single-breath DLCO

The single-breath DLCO test is the most commonly used method for measuring the diffusion capacity of the lungs. This test involves the patient inhaling a gas mixture containing a small amount of CO and a tracer gas (usually helium or methane), holding their breath for a brief period, and then exhaling into a spirometer. The spirometer measures the concentration of CO in the exhaled air, which is used to calculate the amount of CO absorbed into the blood during the breath-hold phase.

Step-by-step Process for SB-DLCO

- *Inhalation of gas mixture*: The patient inhales a known concentration of CO and tracer gas (usually helium) to total lung capacity (TLC).
- *Breath hold*: The patient holds their breath for 10 seconds, allowing the CO to diffuse across the alveolar-capillary membrane into the bloodstream.
- *Exhalation and analysis*: The patient exhales into a spirometer, which measures the concentration of CO in the exhaled air.
- *Calculation*: The DLCO value is calculated based on the reduction in CO concentration in the exhaled air compared to the inhaled concentration. Adjustments are made for alveolar volume (VA) and other factors to derive the final DLCO value.

The SB-DLCO method is the gold standard for measuring DLCO because it provides precise and accurate measurements, allowing for a direct assessment of lung diffusion capacity.

FACTORS AFFECTING DLCO MEASUREMENT

Hemoglobin Concentration

Because CO binds to hemoglobin in the blood, the concentration of hemoglobin directly influences DLCO readings. Anemia, a condition characterized by low hemoglobin levels, can lead to a reduction in DLCO, even in the absence of lung disease. This is because less hemoglobin is available to bind to CO, reducing the measured diffusion capacity.

On the other hand, polycythemia, an increase in red blood cell mass, can lead to an artificially elevated DLCO due to a larger pool of hemoglobin available to bind CO.

Body Position

DLCO can be influenced by the body position in which the test is performed. When the patient is in the supine position, the perfusion of the lungs is typically more uniform, which can lead to higher DLCO values compared to the seated position. The changes in pulmonary blood flow when transitioning from sitting to lying down can affect the interpretation of results, especially in patients with cardiovascular or pulmonary conditions.

Age and Gender

Both age and gender have a significant impact on DLCO values. DLCO generally declines with age due to physiological changes in the lung, such as reduced surface area for gas exchange and decreased pulmonary capillary blood volume. Furthermore, women typically have lower DLCO values than men, primarily due to differences in lung size and blood volume.

Pulmonary Pathologies

The presence of various pulmonary pathologies, such as pulmonary fibrosis, emphysema, or pulmonary vascular disease, can significantly alter DLCO measurements. For instance, in emphysema, the loss of alveolar surface area results in a reduced DLCO, while in pulmonary hypertension, a decrease in pulmonary capillary blood volume leads to a similar decline in DLCO.

CONCLUSION

DLCO is an invaluable tool in modern pulmonary medicine, offering detailed insights into lung function beyond what can be assessed with spirometry. By evaluating the diffusion of gases across the alveolar-capillary membrane, DLCO helps in diagnosing and monitoring a wide range of pulmonary conditions, including ILDs, COPD, pulmonary hypertension, and more.

DLCO testing plays a critical role in the early detection of diseases that affect lung diffusion capacity, such as pulmonary fibrosis, and is essential for assessing the severity and progression of these conditions. Moreover, it is increasingly used to assess the impact of treatment and interventions on pulmonary function, particularly in complex cases involving multiple pulmonary pathologies.

As technology improves and more refined methods of DLCO testing emerge, the role of DLCO in clinical practice will only expand, offering more precise diagnostic information and better management strategies.

Index

L

M

N

O

P

Q

R